This Book Belongs To:

TypeOneToddler.com

Emergency Contacts

Type One Toddler

M T W TH F S SU

Date: / /

Shot Location

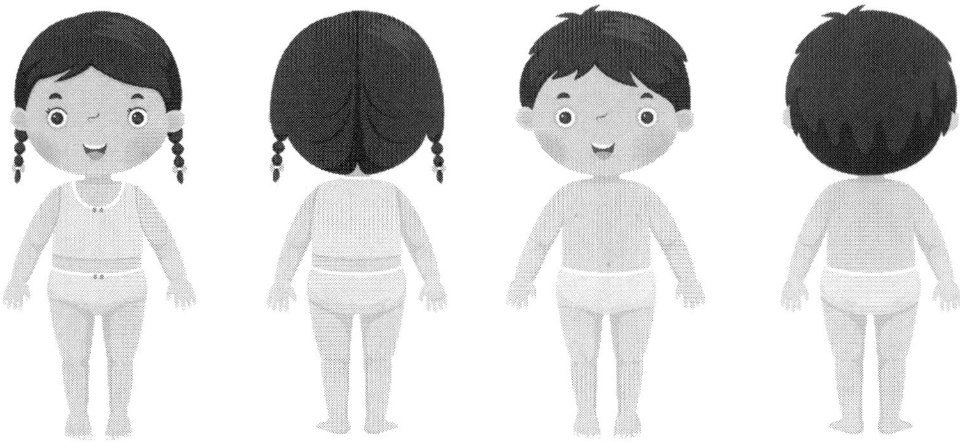

Notes

M T W TH F S SU

Date: / /

	Time	Blood Sugar	Carbs	Insulin	Notes
Breakfast					
Snack					
Lunch					
Snack					
Dinner					
Bedtime					
Night					

M T W TH F S SU Date: / /

Shot Location

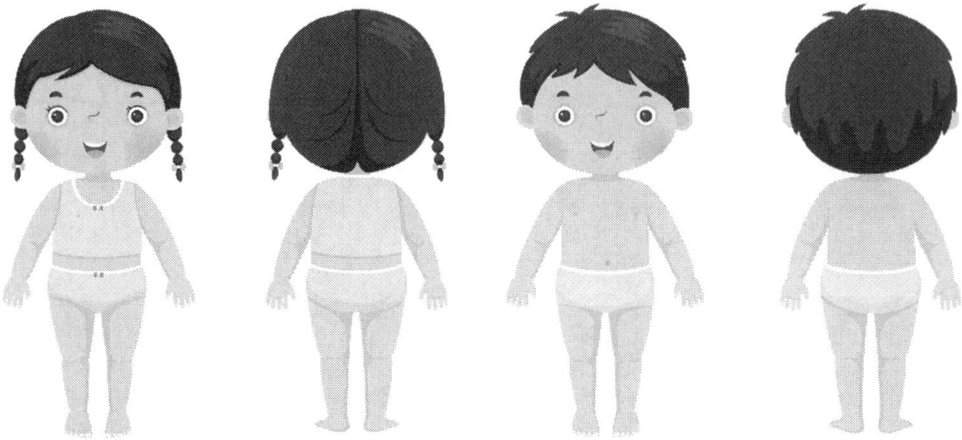

Notes

M T W TH F S SU

Date: / /

	Time	Blood Sugar	Carbs	Insulin	Notes
Breakfast					
Snack					
Lunch					
Snack					
Dinner					
Bedtime					
Night					

M T W TH F S SU Date: / /

Shot Location

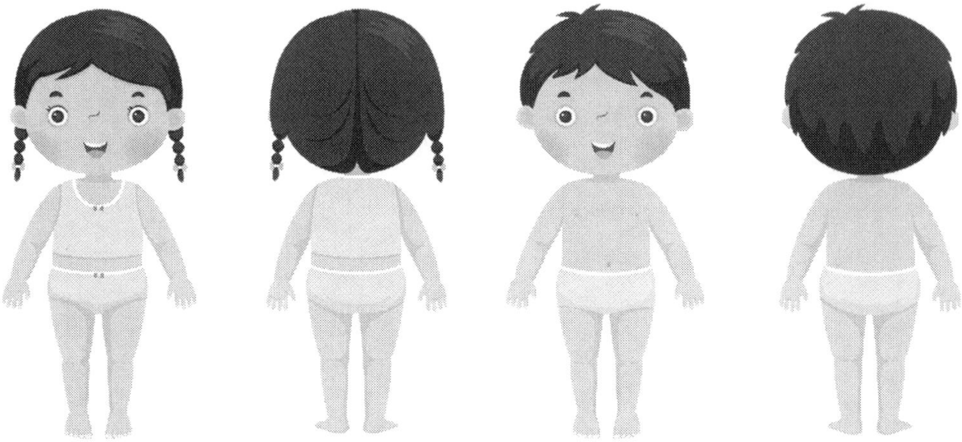

Notes

M T W TH F S SU

Date: / /

	Time	Blood Sugar	Carbs	Insulin	Notes
Breakfast					
Snack					
Lunch					
Snack					
Dinner					
Bedtime					
Night					

M T W TH F S SU

Date: / /

Shot Location

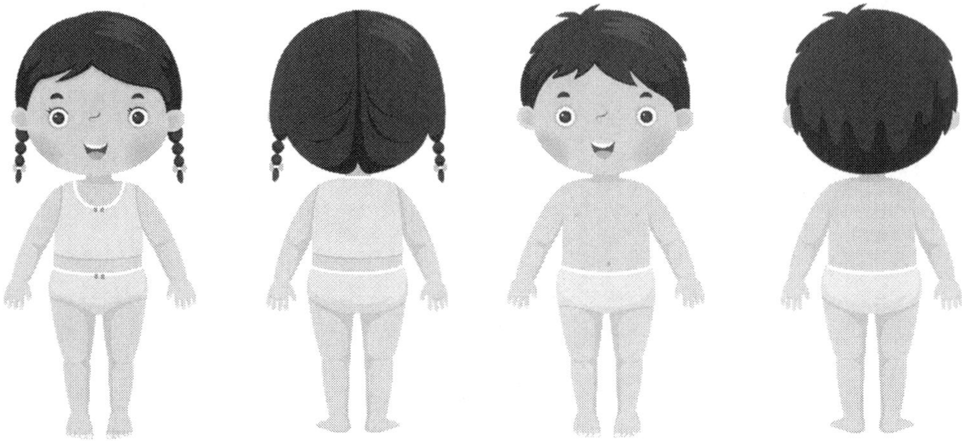

Notes

M T W TH F S SU

Date: / /

	Time	Blood Sugar	Carbs	Insulin	Notes
Breakfast					
Snack					
Lunch					
Snack					
Dinner					
Bedtime					
Night					

M T W TH F S SU Date: / /

Shot Location

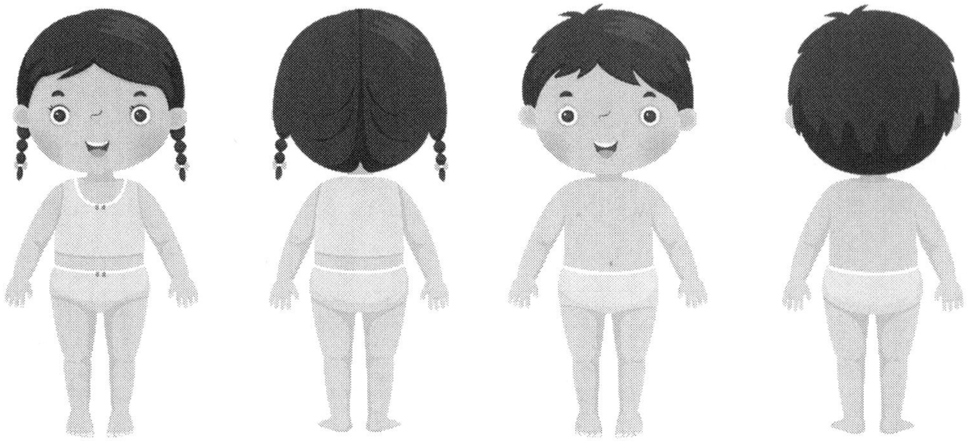

Notes

M T W TH F S SU

Date: / /

	Time	Blood Sugar	Carbs	Insulin	Notes
Breakfast					
Snack					
Lunch					
Snack					
Dinner					
Bedtime					
Night					

M T W TH F S SU

Date: / /

Shot Location

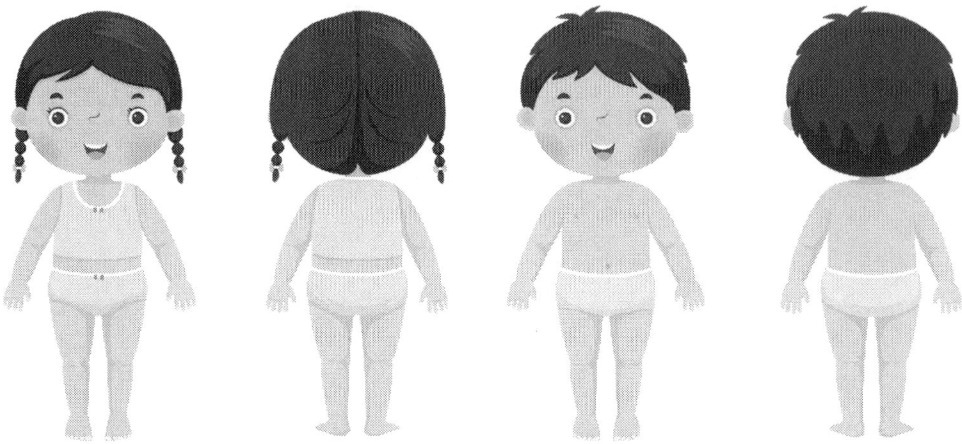

Notes

M T W TH F S SU

Date: / /

	Time	Blood Sugar	Carbs	Insulin	Notes
Breakfast					
Snack					
Lunch					
Snack					
Dinner					
Bedtime					
Night					

M T W TH F S SU Date: / /

Shot Location

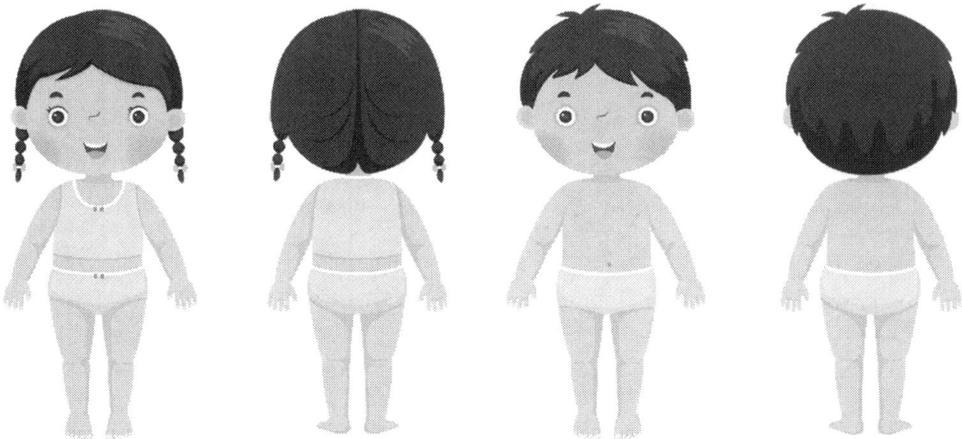

Notes

M T W TH F S SU   Date: / /

	Time	Blood Sugar	Carbs	Insulin	Notes
Breakfast					
Snack					
Lunch					
Snack					
Dinner					
Bedtime					
Night					

M T W TH F S SU Date: / /

Shot Location

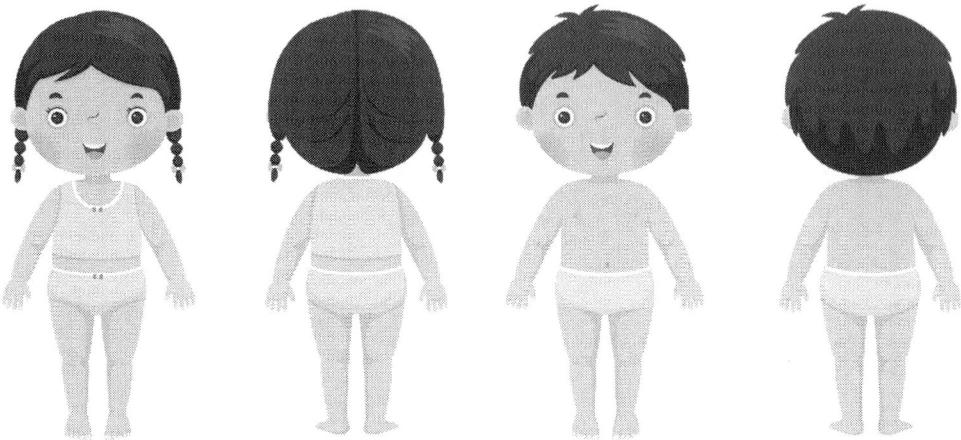

Notes

M T W TH F S SU

Date: / /

	Time	Blood Sugar	Carbs	Insulin	Notes
Breakfast					
Snack					
Lunch					
Snack					
Dinner					
Bedtime					
Night					

M T W TH F S SU Date: / /

Shot Location

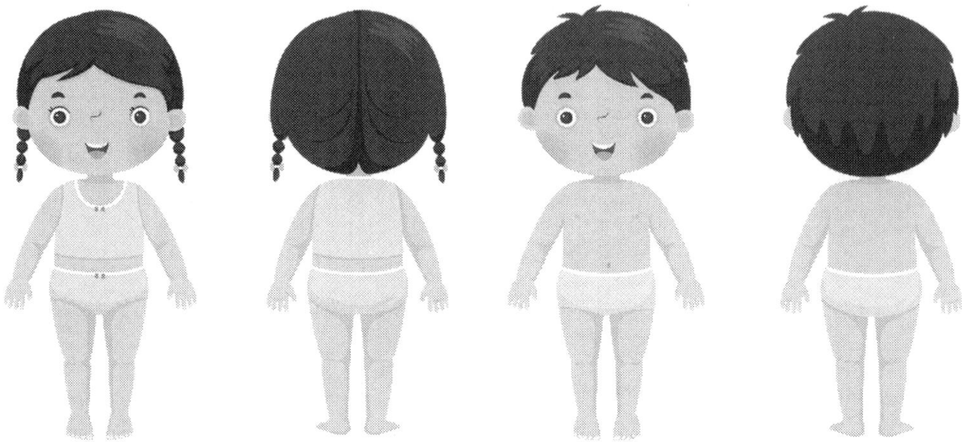

Notes

M T W TH F S SU

Date: / /

	Time	Blood Sugar	Carbs	Insulin	Notes
Breakfast					
Snack					
Lunch					
Snack					
Dinner					
Bedtime					
Night					

M T W TH F S SU Date: / /

Shot Location

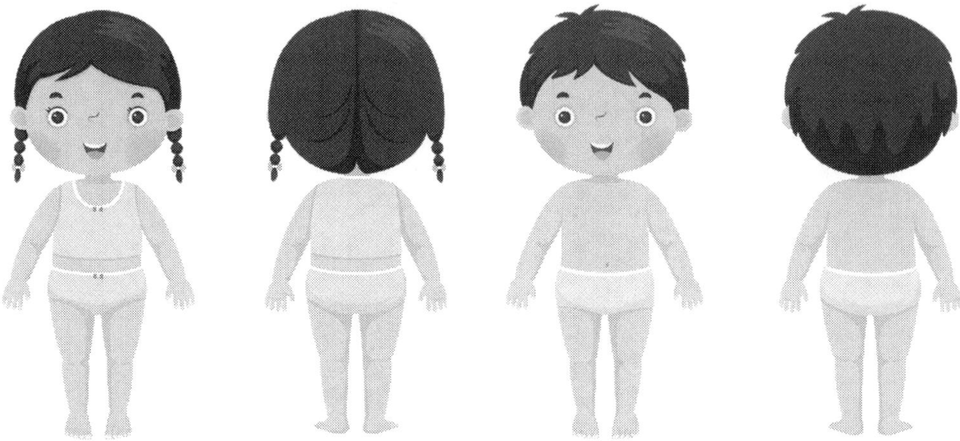

Notes

M T W TH F S SU

Date: / /

	Time	Blood Sugar	Carbs	Insulin	Notes
Breakfast					
Snack					
Lunch					
Snack					
Dinner					
Bedtime					
Night					

M T W TH F S SU Date: / /

Shot Location

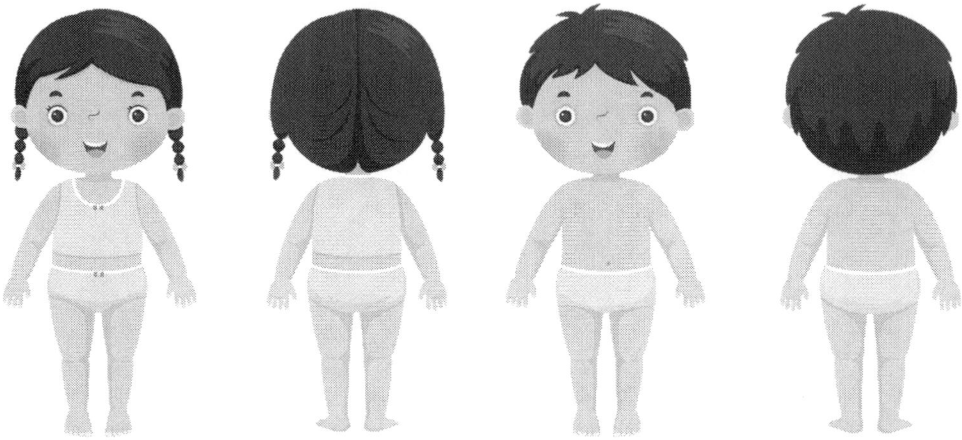

Notes

M T W TH F S SU

Date: / /

	Time	Blood Sugar	Carbs	Insulin	Notes
Breakfast					
Snack					
Lunch					
Snack					
Dinner					
Bedtime					
Night					

M T W TH F S SU Date: / /

Shot Location

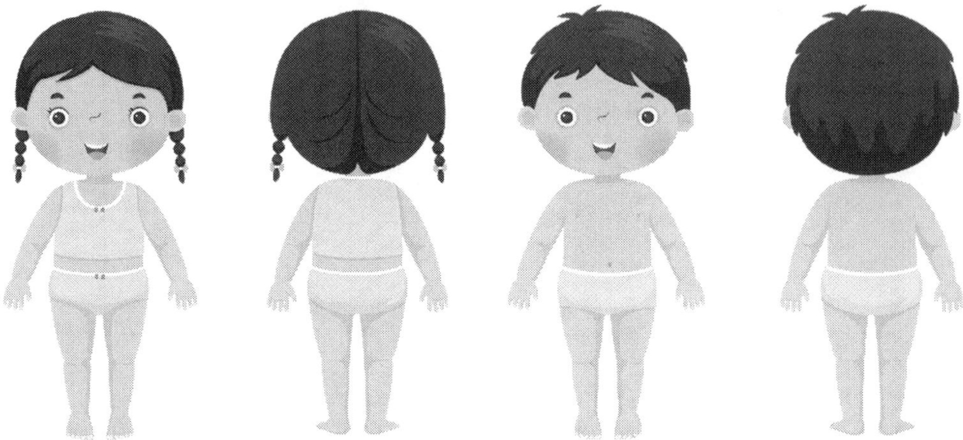

Notes

M T W TH F S SU

Date: / /

	Time	Blood Sugar	Carbs	Insulin	Notes
Breakfast					
Snack					
Lunch					
Snack					
Dinner					
Bedtime					
Night					

M T W TH F S SU Date: / /

Shot Location

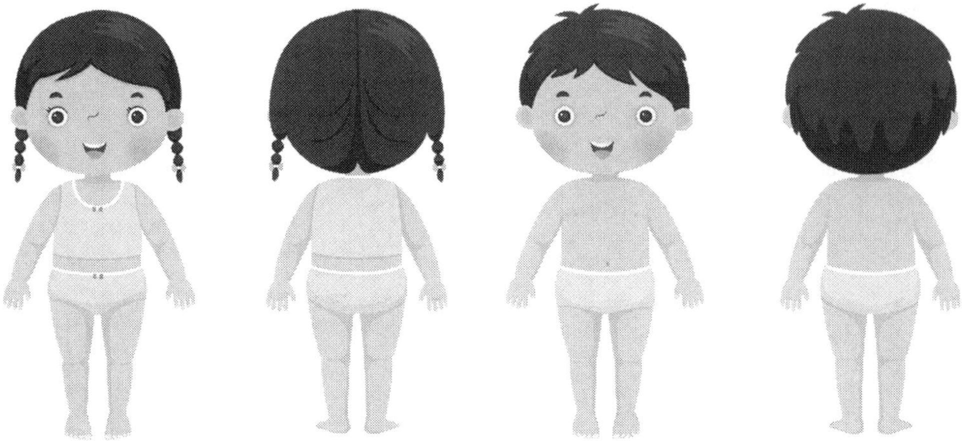

Notes

M T W TH F S SU

Date: / /

	Time	Blood Sugar	Carbs	Insulin	Notes
Breakfast					
Snack					
Lunch					
Snack					
Dinner					
Bedtime					
Night					

M T W TH F S SU Date: / /

Shot Location

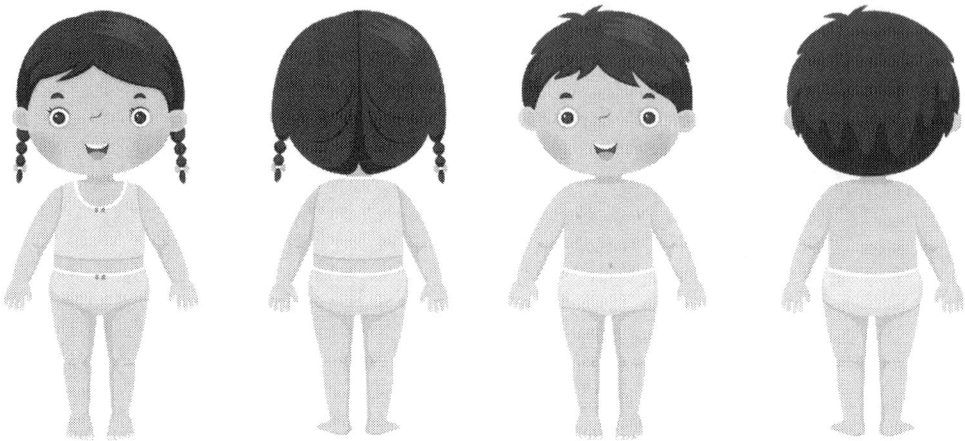

Notes

M T W TH F S SU Date: / /

	Time	Blood Sugar	Carbs	Insulin	Notes
Breakfast					
Snack					
Lunch					
Snack					
Dinner					
Bedtime					
Night					

M T W TH F S SU Date: / /

Shot Location

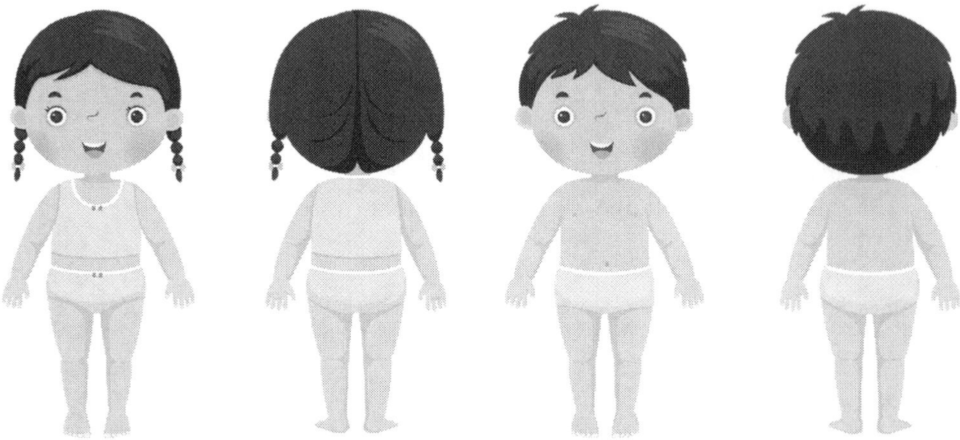

Notes

M T W TH F S SU

Date: / /

	Time	Blood Sugar	Carbs	Insulin	Notes
Breakfast					
Snack					
Lunch					
Snack					
Dinner					
Bedtime					
Night					

M T W TH F S SU

Date: / /

Shot Location

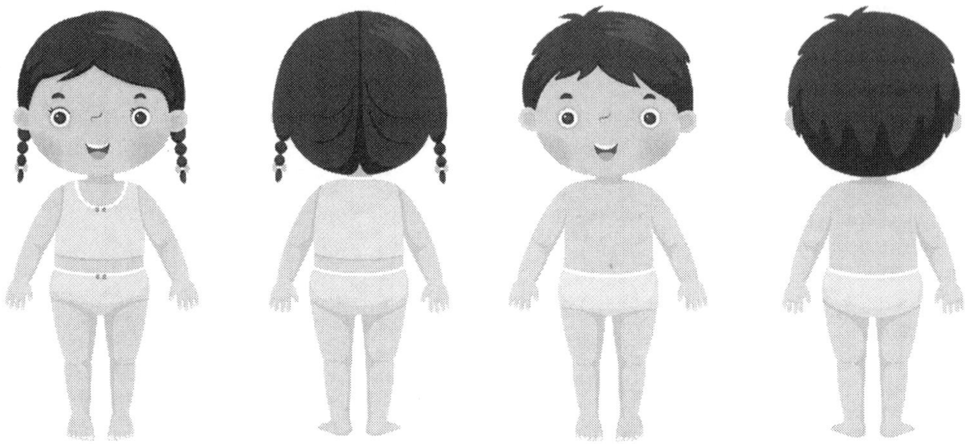

Notes

M T W TH F S SU Date: / /

	Time	Blood Sugar	Carbs	Insulin	Notes
Breakfast					
Snack					
Lunch					
Snack					
Dinner					
Bedtime					
Night					

M T W TH F S SU Date: / /

Shot Location

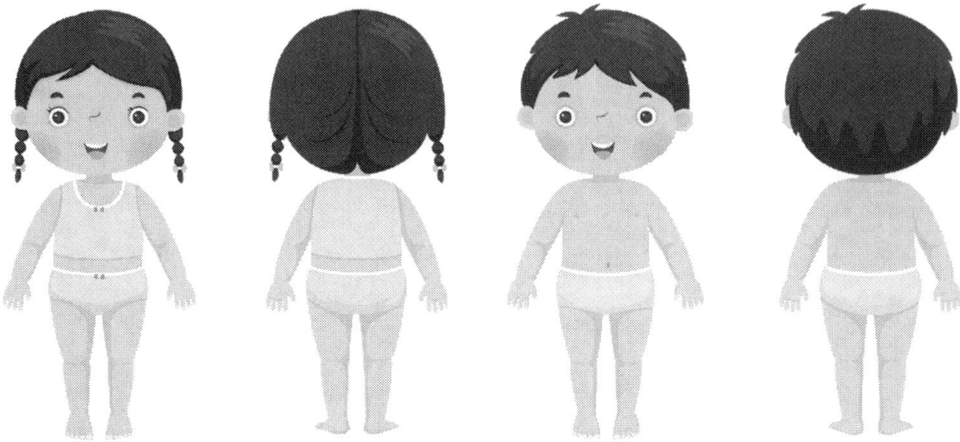

Notes

M T W TH F S SU

Date: / /

	Time	Blood Sugar	Carbs	Insulin	Notes
Breakfast					
Snack					
Lunch					
Snack					
Dinner					
Bedtime					
Night					

M T W TH F S SU Date: / /

Shot Location

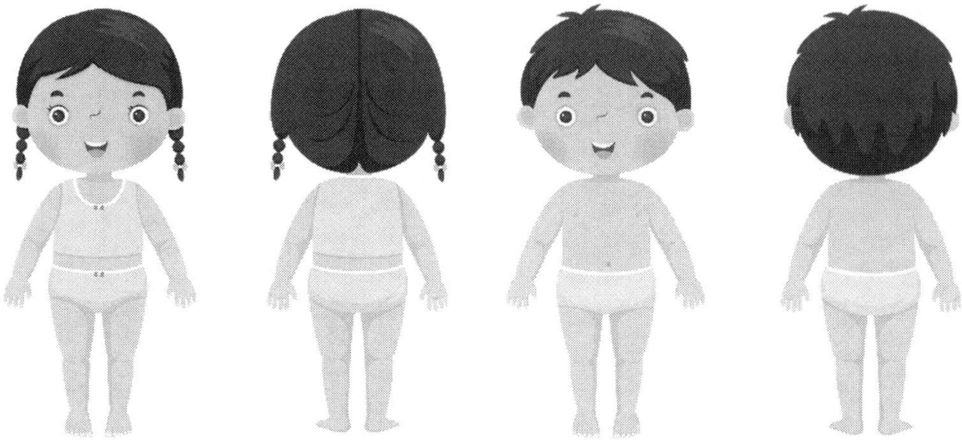

Notes

M T W TH F S SU

Date: / /

	Time	Blood Sugar	Carbs	Insulin	Notes
Breakfast					
Snack					
Lunch					
Snack					
Dinner					
Bedtime					
Night					

M T W TH F S SU Date: / /

Shot Location

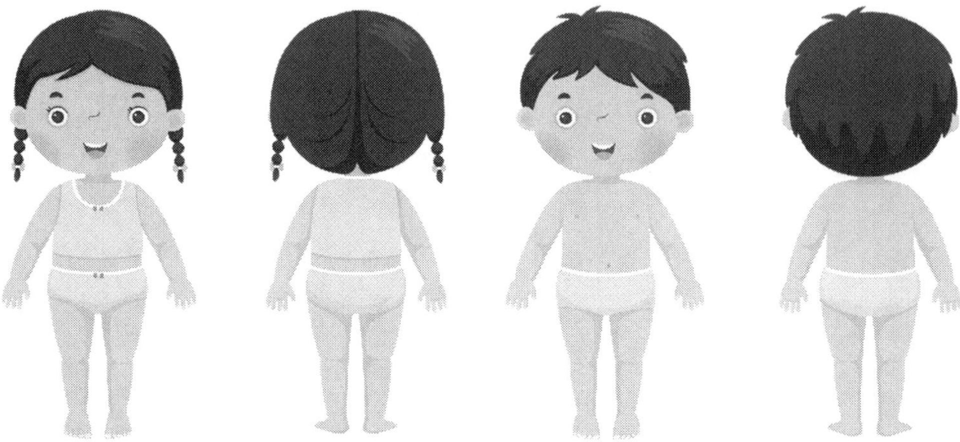

Notes

M T W TH F S SU

Date: / /

	Time	Blood Sugar	Carbs	Insulin	Notes
Breakfast					
Snack					
Lunch					
Snack					
Dinner					
Bedtime					
Night					

M T W TH F S SU

Date: / /

Shot Location

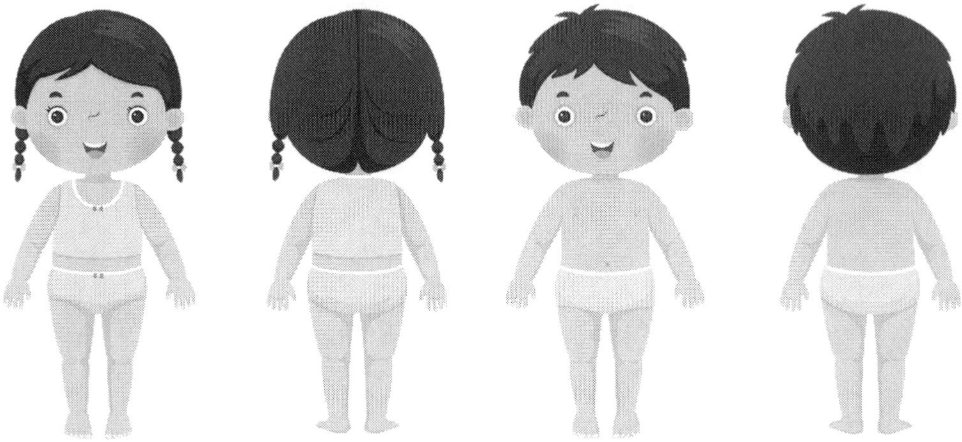

Notes

M T W TH F S SU

Date: / /

	Time	Blood Sugar	Carbs	Insulin	Notes
Breakfast					
Snack					
Lunch					
Snack					
Dinner					
Bedtime					
Night					

M T W TH F S SU   Date: / /

Shot Location

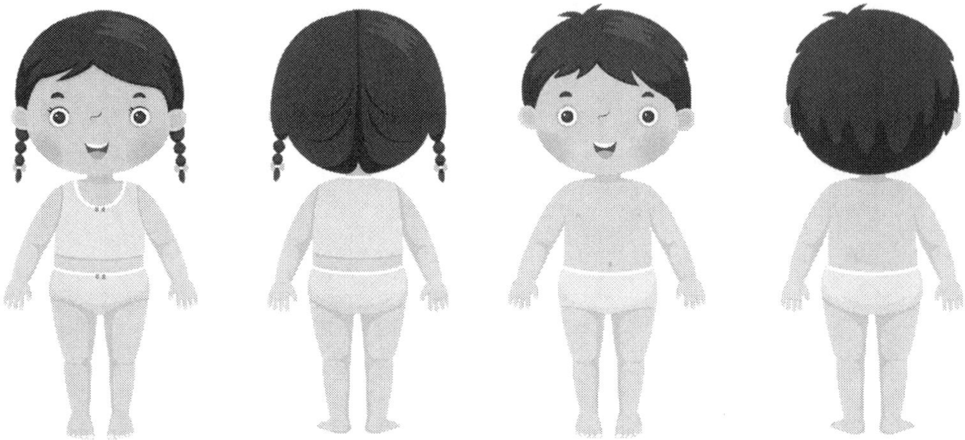

Notes

M T W TH F S SU

Date: / /

	Time	Blood Sugar	Carbs	Insulin	Notes
Breakfast					
Snack					
Lunch					
Snack					
Dinner					
Bedtime					
Night					

M T W TH F S SU Date: / /

Shot Location

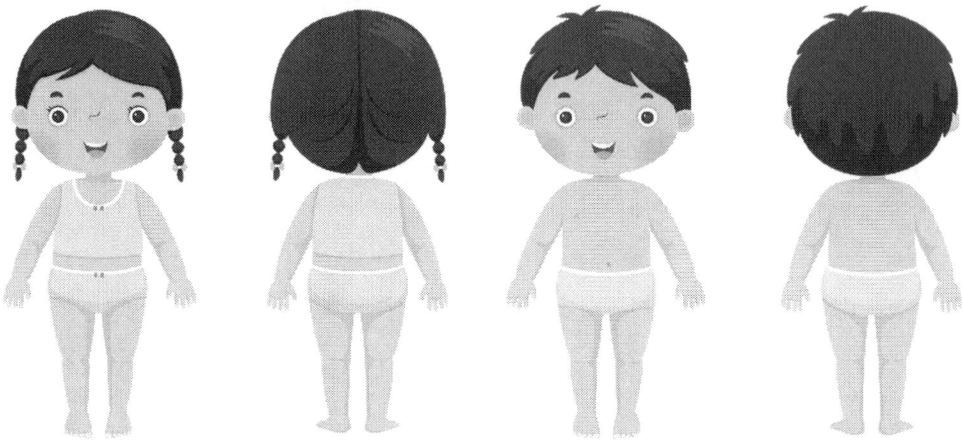

Notes

M T W TH F S SU

Date: / /

	Time	Blood Sugar	Carbs	Insulin	Notes
Breakfast					
Snack					
Lunch					
Snack					
Dinner					
Bedtime					
Night					

M T W TH F S SU Date: / /

Shot Location

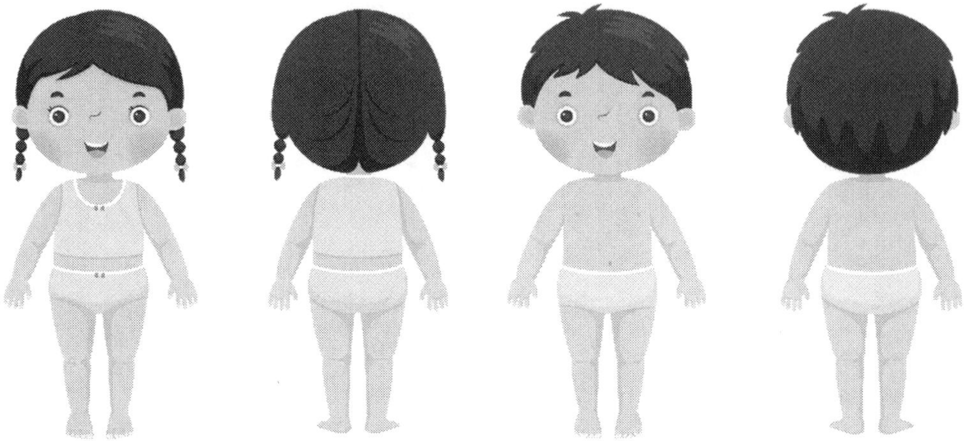

Notes

M T W TH F S SU

Date: / /

	Time	Blood Sugar	Carbs	Insulin	Notes
Breakfast					
Snack					
Lunch					
Snack					
Dinner					
Bedtime					
Night					

M T W TH F S SU Date: / /

Shot Location

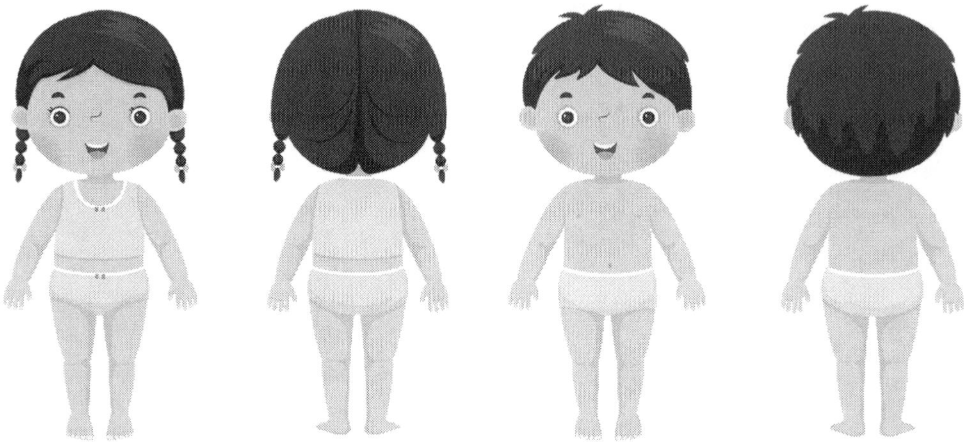

Notes

M T W TH F S SU

Date: / /

	Time	Blood Sugar	Carbs	Insulin	Notes
Breakfast					
Snack					
Lunch					
Snack					
Dinner					
Bedtime					
Night					

M T W TH F S SU Date: / /

Shot Location

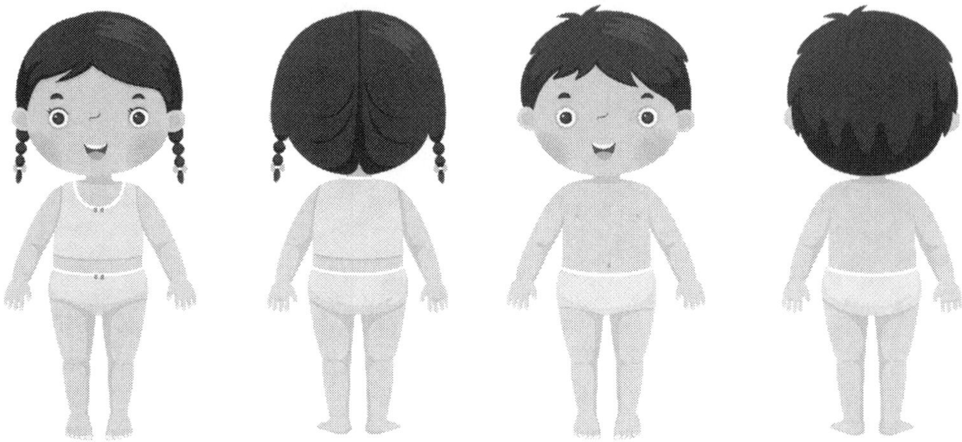

Notes

M T W TH F S SU

Date: / /

	Time	Blood Sugar	Carbs	Insulin	Notes
Breakfast					
Snack					
Lunch					
Snack					
Dinner					
Bedtime					
Night					

M T W TH F S SU Date: / /

Shot Location

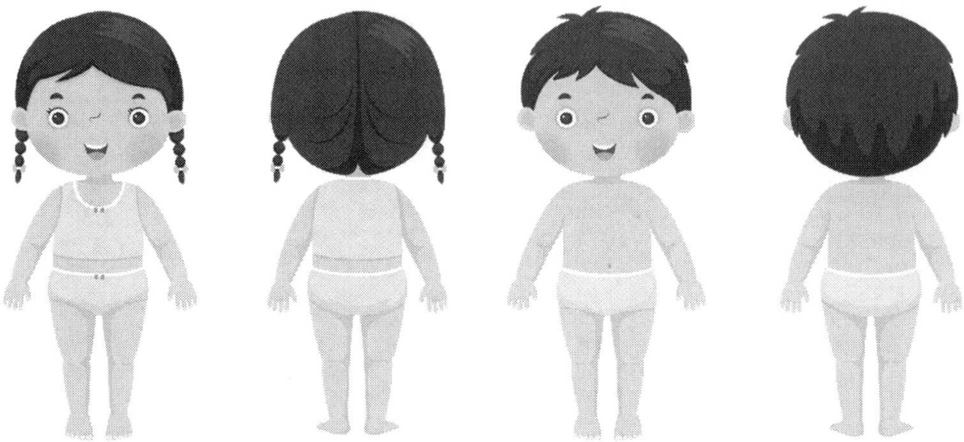

Notes

M T W TH F S SU

Date: / /

	Time	Blood Sugar	Carbs	Insulin	Notes
Breakfast					
Snack					
Lunch					
Snack					
Dinner					
Bedtime					
Night					

M T W TH F S SU Date: / /

Shot Location

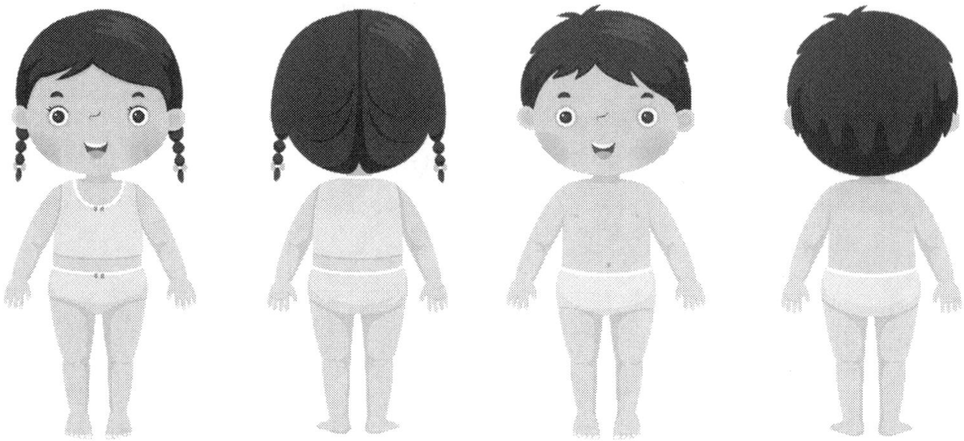

Notes

M T W TH F S SU

Date: / /

	Time	Blood Sugar	Carbs	Insulin	Notes
Breakfast					
Snack					
Lunch					
Snack					
Dinner					
Bedtime					
Night					

M T W TH F S SU Date: / /

Shot Location

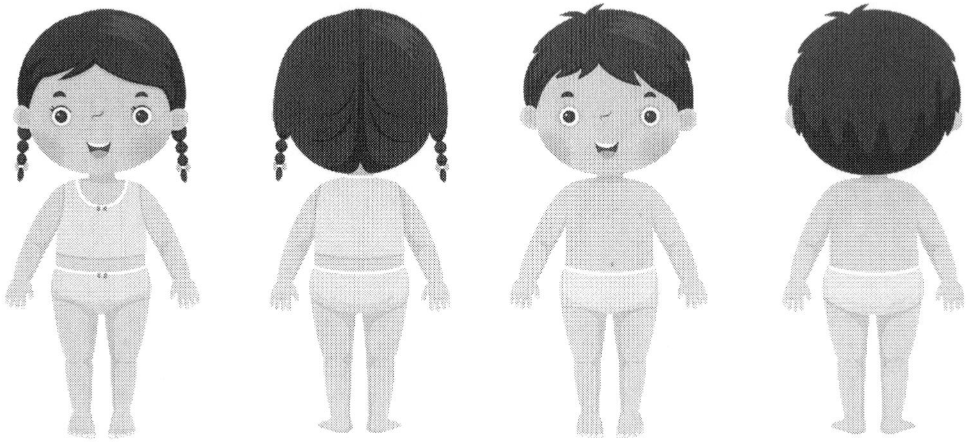

Notes

M T W TH F S SU

Date: / /

	Time	Blood Sugar	Carbs	Insulin	Notes
Breakfast					
Snack					
Lunch					
Snack					
Dinner					
Bedtime					
Night					

M T W TH F S SU Date: / /

Shot Location

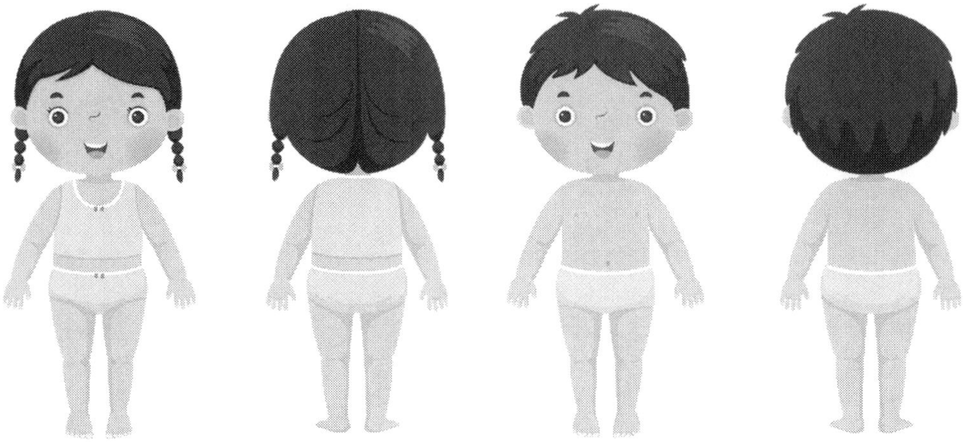

Notes

M T W TH F S SU

Date: / /

	Time	Blood Sugar	Carbs	Insulin	Notes
Breakfast					
Snack					
Lunch					
Snack					
Dinner					
Bedtime					
Night					

M T W TH F S SU Date: / /

Shot Location

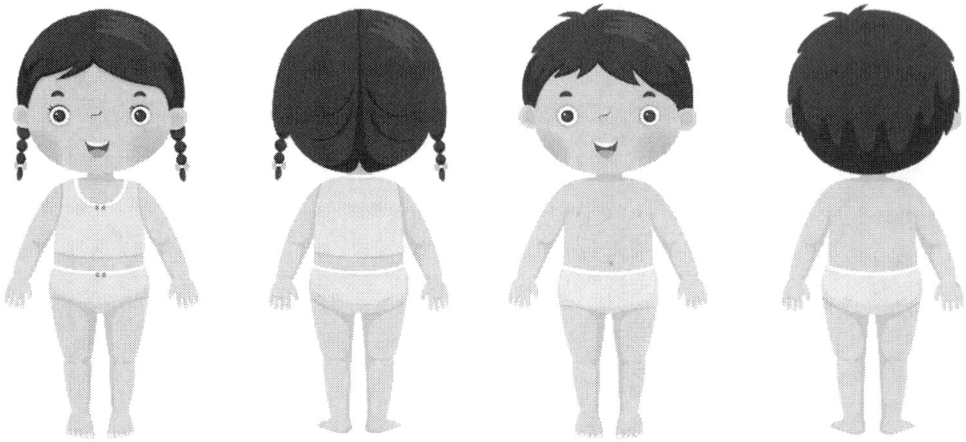

Notes

M T W TH F S SU

Date: / /

	Time	Blood Sugar	Carbs	Insulin	Notes
Breakfast					
Snack					
Lunch					
Snack					
Dinner					
Bedtime					
Night					

M T W TH F S SU Date: / /

Shot Location

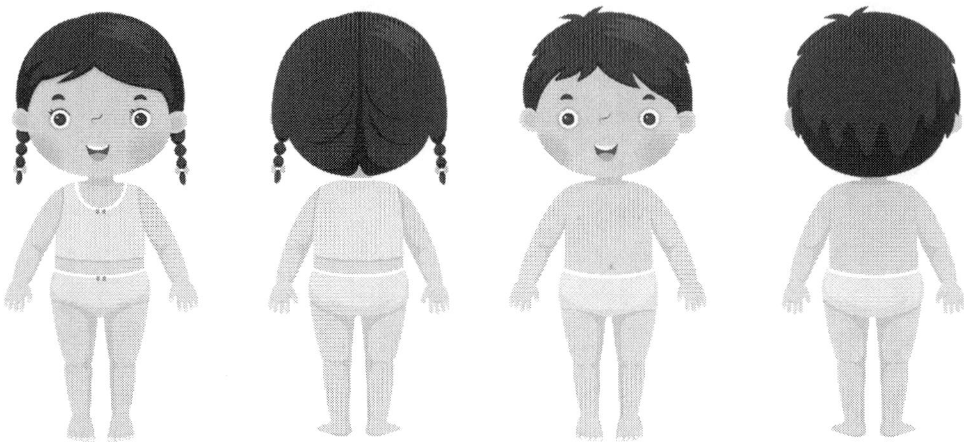

Notes

M T W TH F S SU

Date: / /

	Time	Blood Sugar	Carbs	Insulin	Notes
Breakfast					
Snack					
Lunch					
Snack					
Dinner					
Bedtime					
Night					

M T W TH F S SU Date: / /

Shot Location

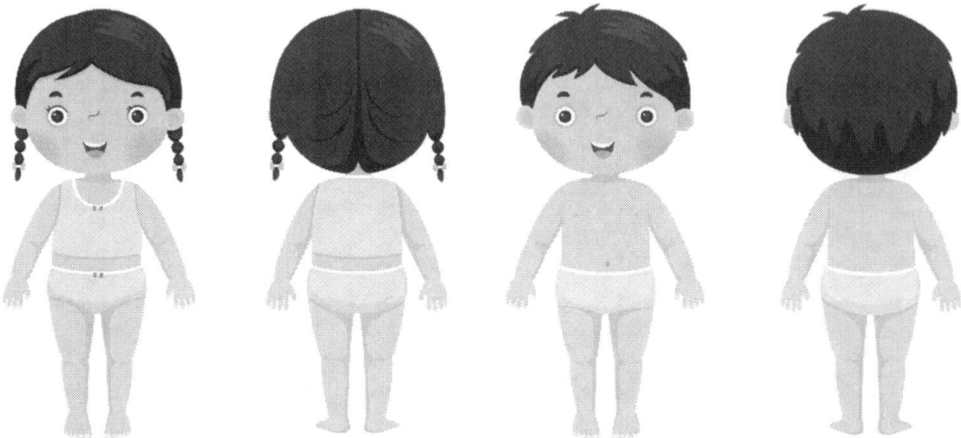

Notes

M T W TH F S SU

Date: / /

	Time	Blood Sugar	Carbs	Insulin	Notes
Breakfast					
Snack					
Lunch					
Snack					
Dinner					
Bedtime					
Night					

M T W TH F S SU Date: / /

Shot Location

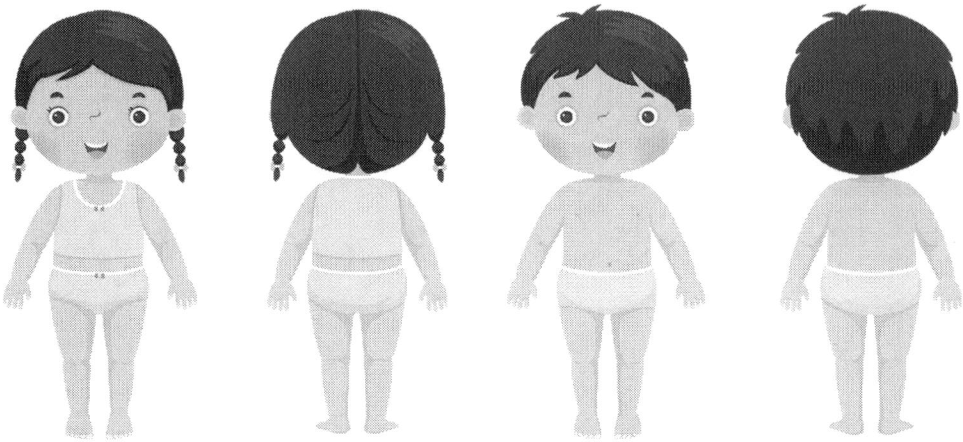

Notes

M T W TH F S SU Date: / /

	Time	Blood Sugar	Carbs	Insulin	Notes
Breakfast					
Snack					
Lunch					
Snack					
Dinner					
Bedtime					
Night					

M T W TH F S SU Date: / /

Shot Location

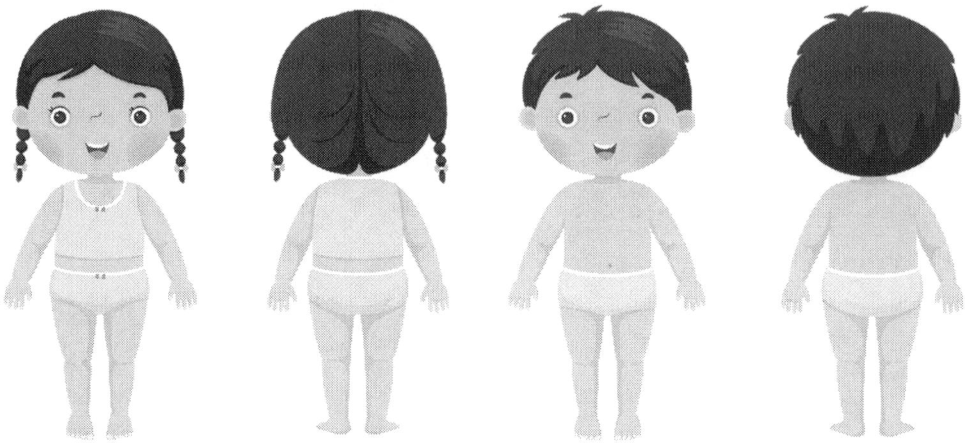

Notes

M T W TH F S SU Date: / /

	Time	Blood Sugar	Carbs	Insulin	Notes
Breakfast					
Snack					
Lunch					
Snack					
Dinner					
Bedtime					
Night					

M T W TH F S SU Date: / /

Shot Location

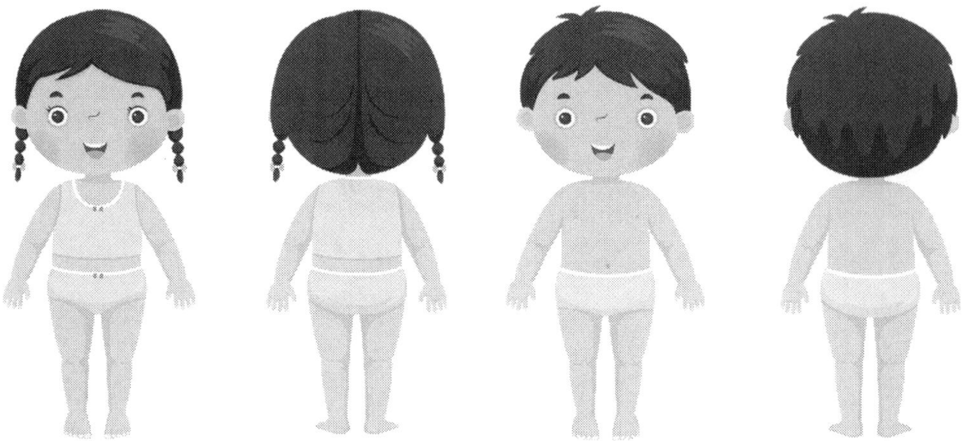

Notes

M T W TH F S SU

Date: / /

	Time	Blood Sugar	Carbs	Insulin	Notes
Breakfast					
Snack					
Lunch					
Snack					
Dinner					
Bedtime					
Night					

M T W TH F S SU Date: / /

Shot Location

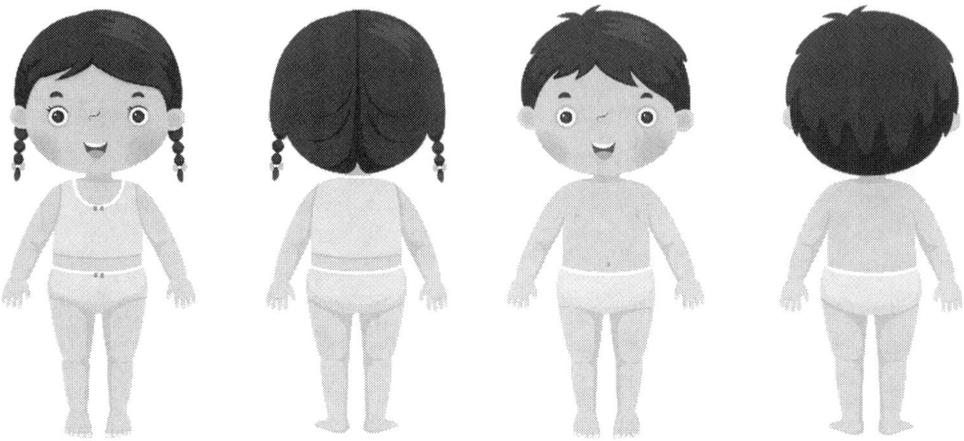

Notes

M T W TH F S SU

Date: / /

	Time	Blood Sugar	Carbs	Insulin	Notes
Breakfast					
Snack					
Lunch					
Snack					
Dinner					
Bedtime					
Night					

M T W TH F S SU

Date: / /

Shot Location

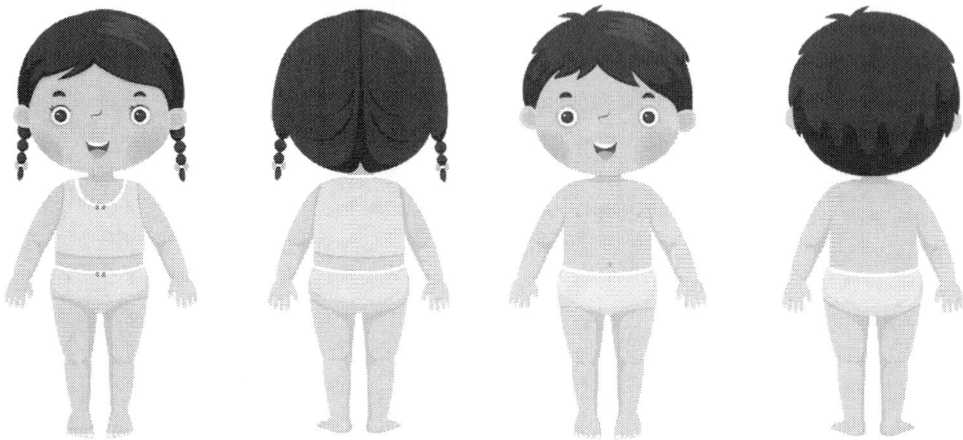

Notes

M T W TH F S SU

Date: / /

	Time	Blood Sugar	Carbs	Insulin	Notes
Breakfast					
Snack					
Lunch					
Snack					
Dinner					
Bedtime					
Night					

M T W TH F S SU Date: / /

Shot Location

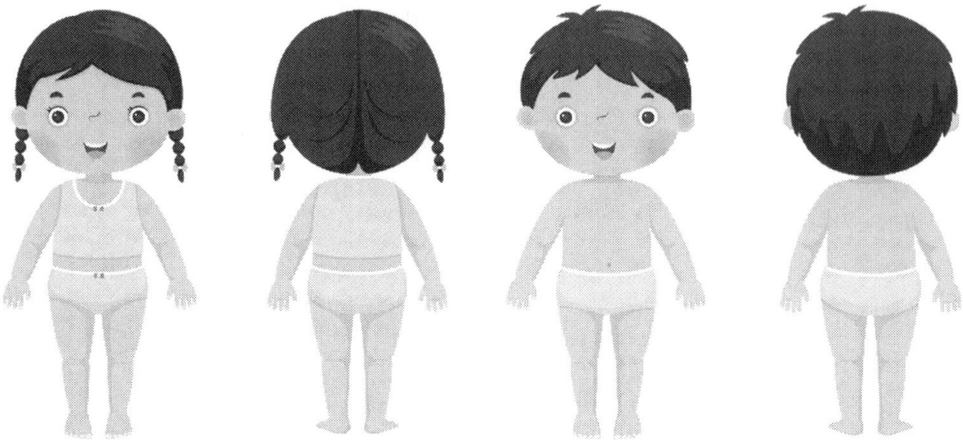

Notes

M T W TH F S SU

Date: / /

	Time	Blood Sugar	Carbs	Insulin	Notes
Breakfast					
Snack					
Lunch					
Snack					
Dinner					
Bedtime					
Night					

M T W TH F S SU Date: / /

Shot Location

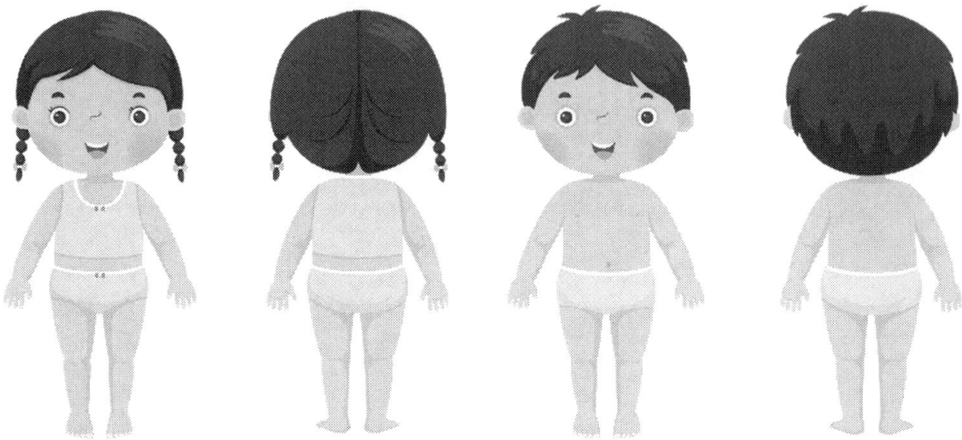

Notes

M T W TH F S SU

Date: / /

	Time	Blood Sugar	Carbs	Insulin	Notes
Breakfast					
Snack					
Lunch					
Snack					
Dinner					
Bedtime					
Night					

M T W TH F S SU Date: / /

Shot Location

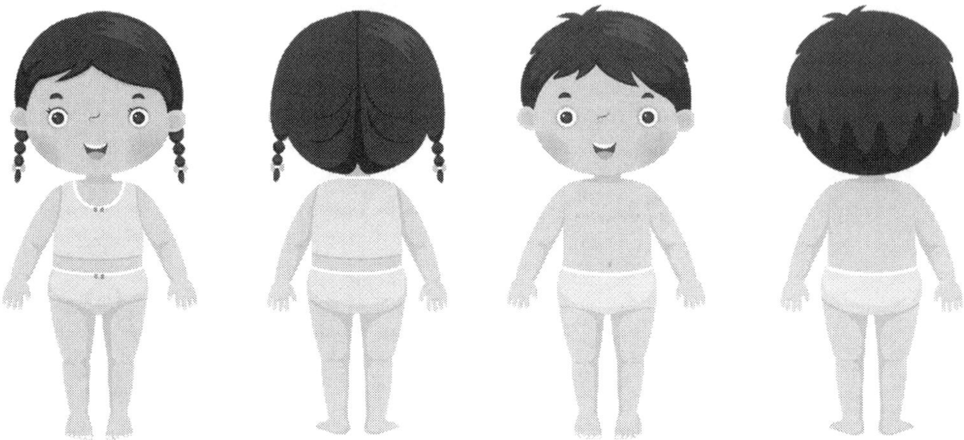

Notes

M T W TH F S SU

Date: / /

	Time	Blood Sugar	Carbs	Insulin	Notes
Breakfast					
Snack					
Lunch					
Snack					
Dinner					
Bedtime					
Night					

M T W TH F S SU Date: / /

Shot Location

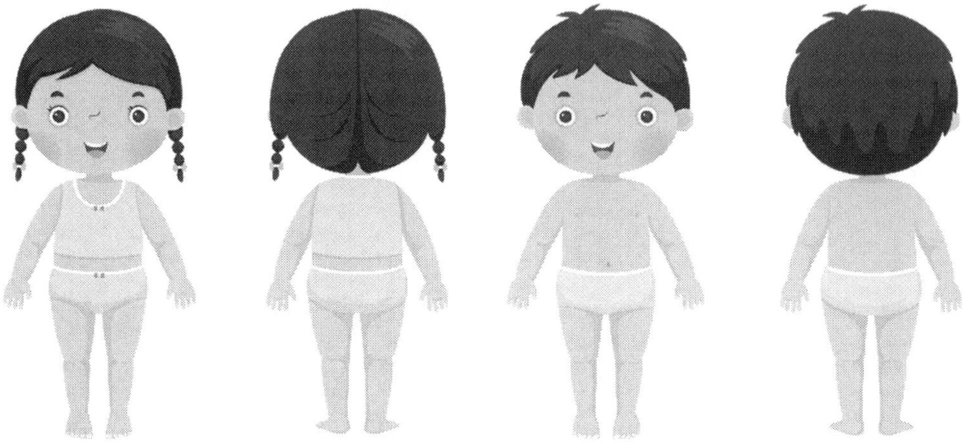

Notes

M T W TH F S SU

Date: / /

	Time	Blood Sugar	Carbs	Insulin	Notes
Breakfast					
Snack					
Lunch					
Snack					
Dinner					
Bedtime					
Night					

M T W TH F S SU

Date: / /

Shot Location

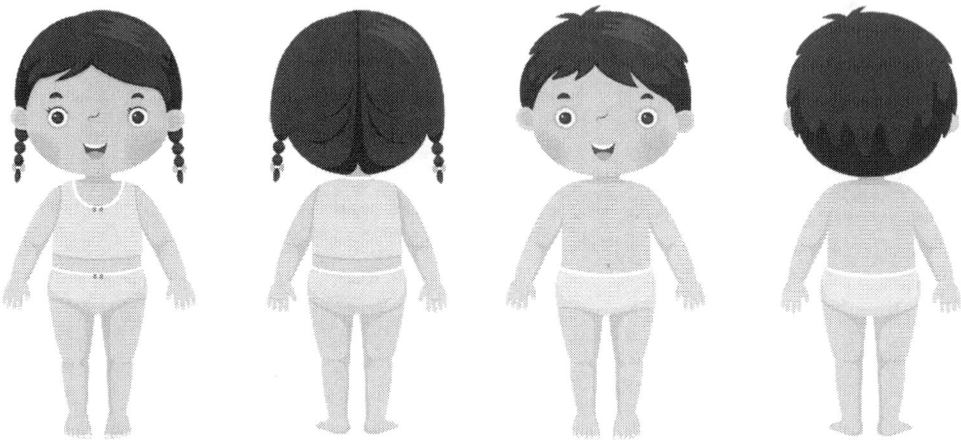

Notes

M T W TH F S SU

Date: / /

	Time	Blood Sugar	Carbs	Insulin	Notes
Breakfast					
Snack					
Lunch					
Snack					
Dinner					
Bedtime					
Night					

M T W TH F S SU Date: / /

Shot Location

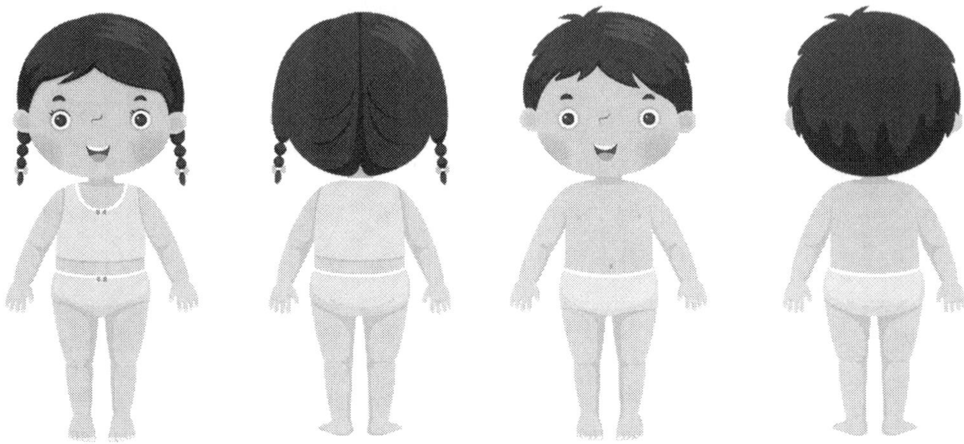

Notes

M T W TH F S SU

Date: / /

	Time	Blood Sugar	Carbs	Insulin	Notes
Breakfast					
Snack					
Lunch					
Snack					
Dinner					
Bedtime					
Night					

M T W TH F S SU

Date: / /

Shot Location

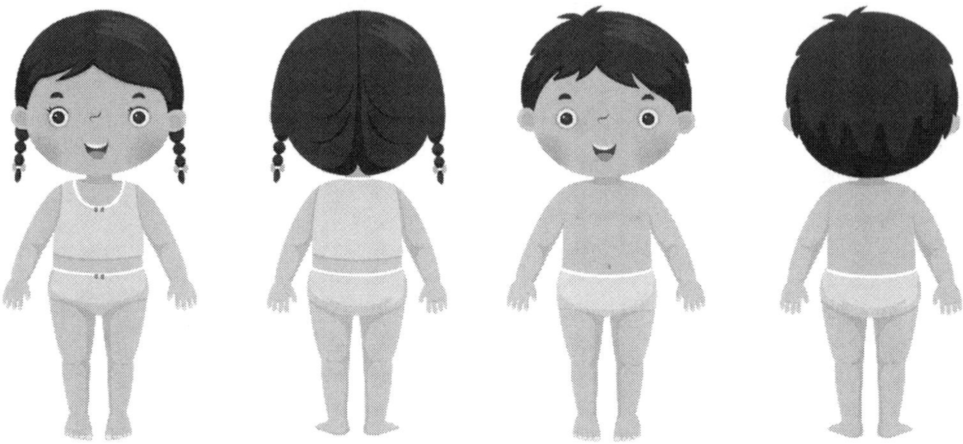

Notes

M T W TH F S SU

Date: / /

	Time	Blood Sugar	Carbs	Insulin	Notes
Breakfast					
Snack					
Lunch					
Snack					
Dinner					
Bedtime					
Night					

M T W TH F S SU Date: / /

Shot Location

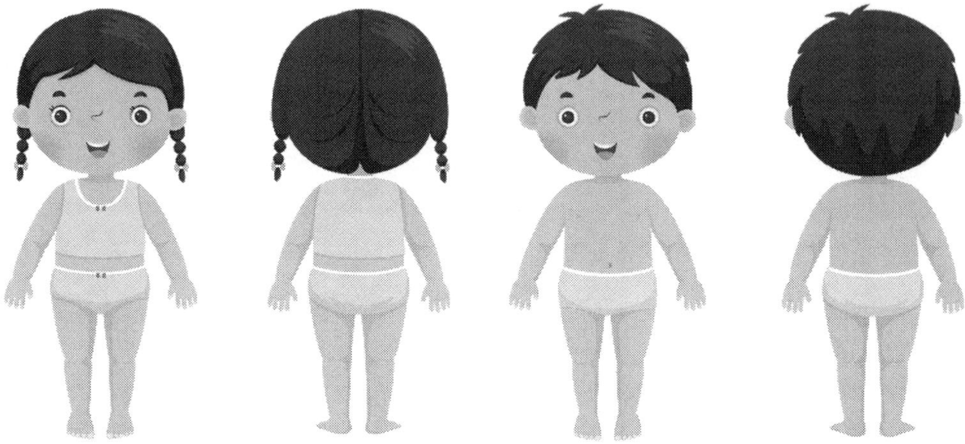

Notes

M T W TH F S SU

Date: / /

	Time	Blood Sugar	Carbs	Insulin	Notes
Breakfast					
Snack					
Lunch					
Snack					
Dinner					
Bedtime					
Night					

M T W TH F S SU Date: / /

Shot Location

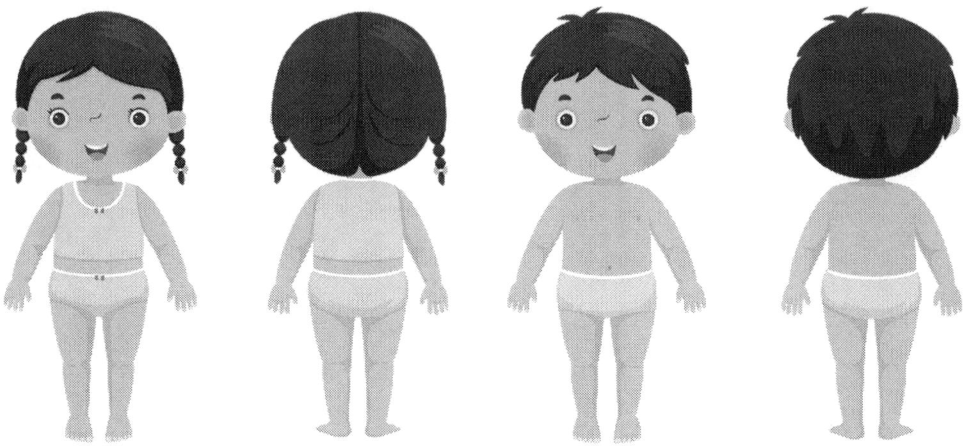

Notes

M T W TH F S SU

Date: / /

	Time	Blood Sugar	Carbs	Insulin	Notes
Breakfast					
Snack					
Lunch					
Snack					
Dinner					
Bedtime					
Night					

M T W TH F S SU Date: / /

Shot Location

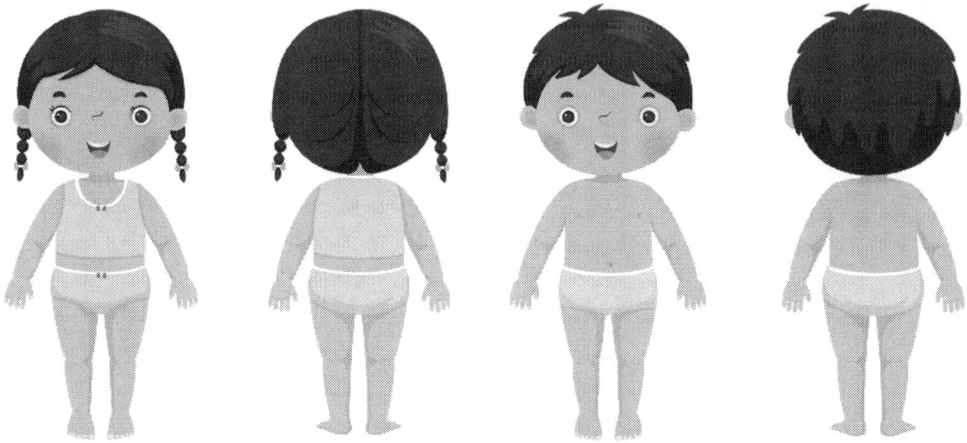

Notes

M T W TH F S SU

Date: / /

	Time	Blood Sugar	Carbs	Insulin	Notes
Breakfast					
Snack					
Lunch					
Snack					
Dinner					
Bedtime					
Night					

M T W TH F S SU Date: / /

Shot Location

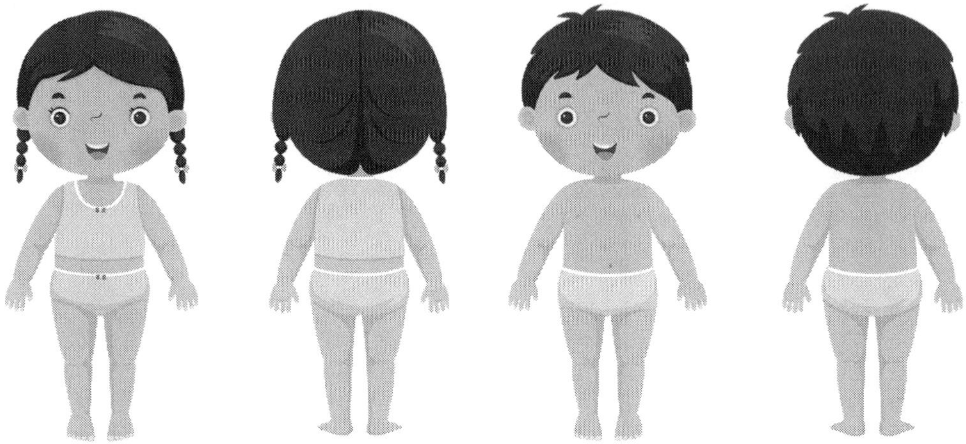

Notes

M T W TH F S SU

Date: / /

	Time	Blood Sugar	Carbs	Insulin	Notes
Breakfast					
Snack					
Lunch					
Snack					
Dinner					
Bedtime					
Night					

M T W TH F S SU

Date: / /

Shot Location

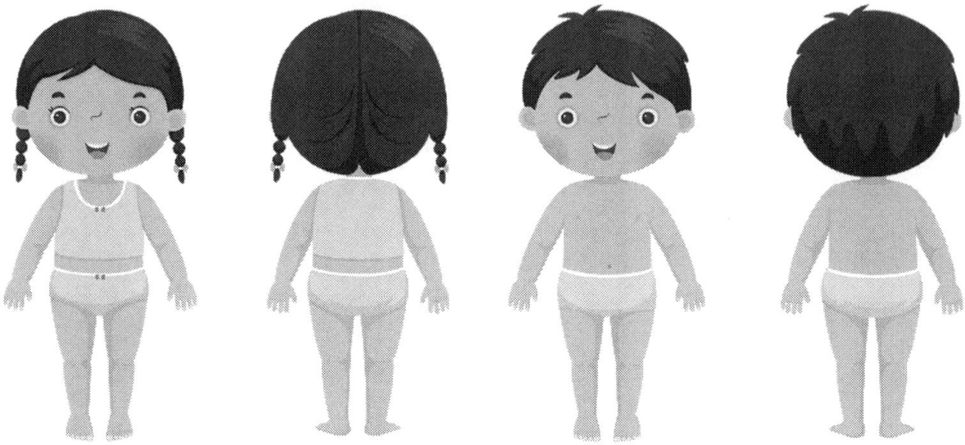

Notes

M T W TH F S SU

Date: / /

	Time	Blood Sugar	Carbs	Insulin	Notes
Breakfast					
Snack					
Lunch					
Snack					
Dinner					
Bedtime					
Night					

M T W TH F S SU Date: / /

Shot Location

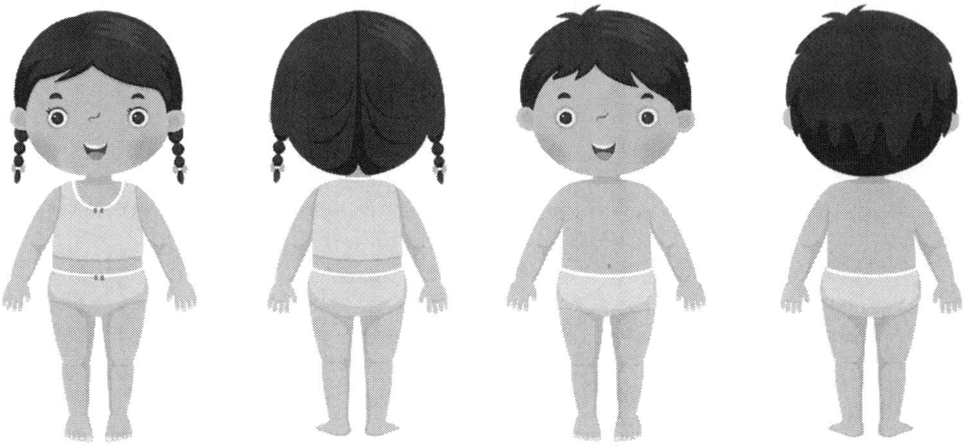

Notes

M T W TH F S SU

Date: / /

	Time	Blood Sugar	Carbs	Insulin	Notes
Breakfast					
Snack					
Lunch					
Snack					
Dinner					
Bedtime					
Night					

M T W TH F S SU

Date: / /

Shot Location

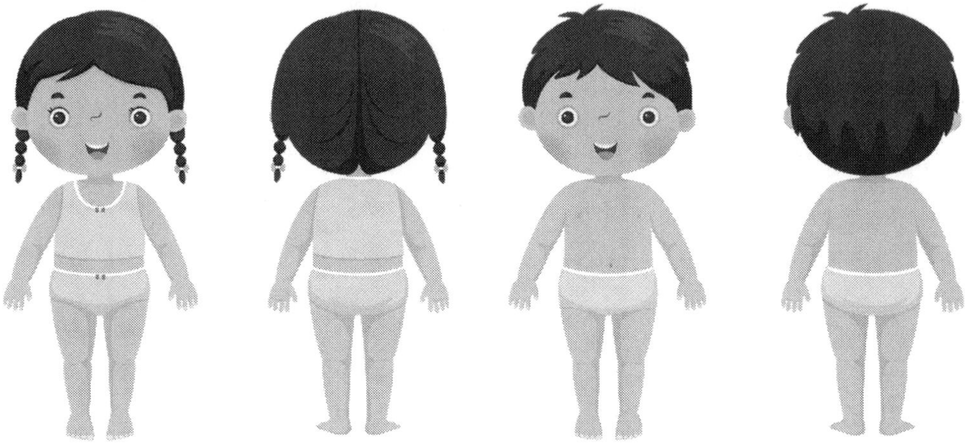

Notes

M T W TH F S SU

Date: / /

	Time	Blood Sugar	Carbs	Insulin	Notes
Breakfast					
Snack					
Lunch					
Snack					
Dinner					
Bedtime					
Night					

M T W TH F S SU Date: / /

Shot Location

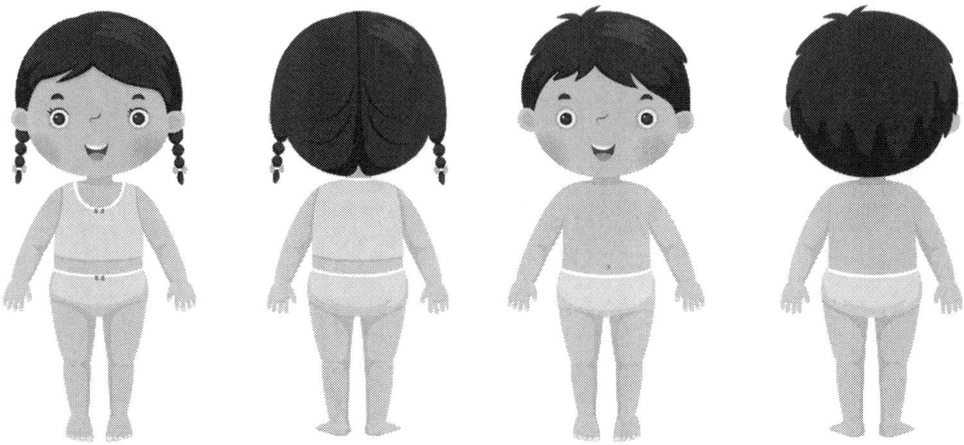

Notes

M T W TH F S SU Date: / /

	Time	Blood Sugar	Carbs	Insulin	Notes
Breakfast					
Snack					
Lunch					
Snack					
Dinner					
Bedtime					
Night					

M T W TH F S SU

Date: / /

Shot Location

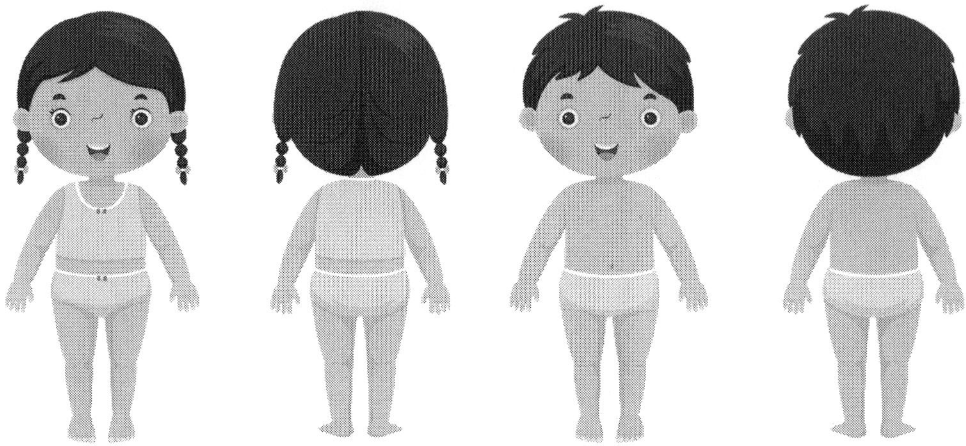

Notes

M T W TH F S SU

Date: / /

	Time	Blood Sugar	Carbs	Insulin	Notes
Breakfast					
Snack					
Lunch					
Snack					
Dinner					
Bedtime					
Night					

M T W TH F S SU Date: / /

Shot Location

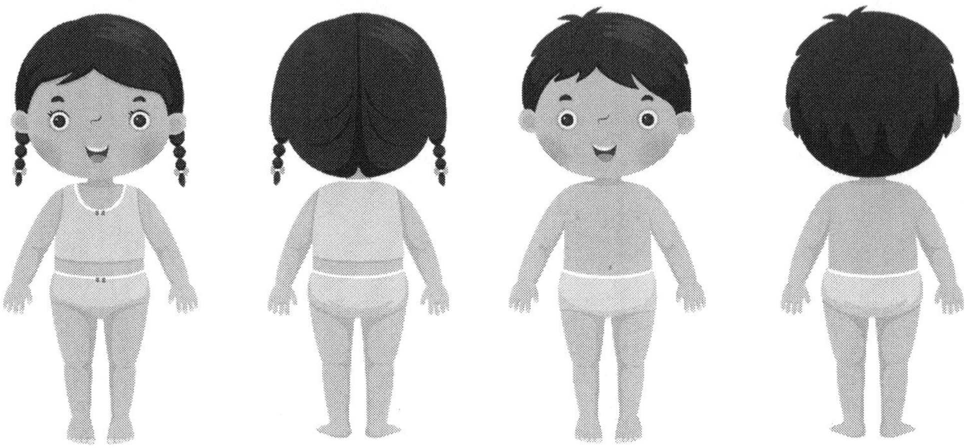

Notes

M T W TH F S SU

Date: / /

	Time	Blood Sugar	Carbs	Insulin	Notes
Breakfast					
Snack					
Lunch					
Snack					
Dinner					
Bedtime					
Night					

M T W TH F S SU Date: / /

Shot Location

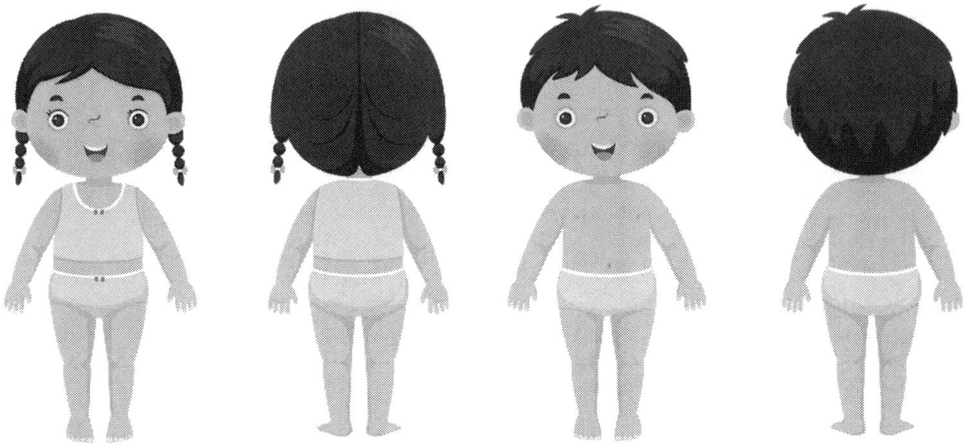

Notes

M T W TH F S SU

Date: / /

	Time	Blood Sugar	Carbs	Insulin	Notes
Breakfast					
Snack					
Lunch					
Snack					
Dinner					
Bedtime					
Night					

M T W TH F S SU Date: / /

Shot Location

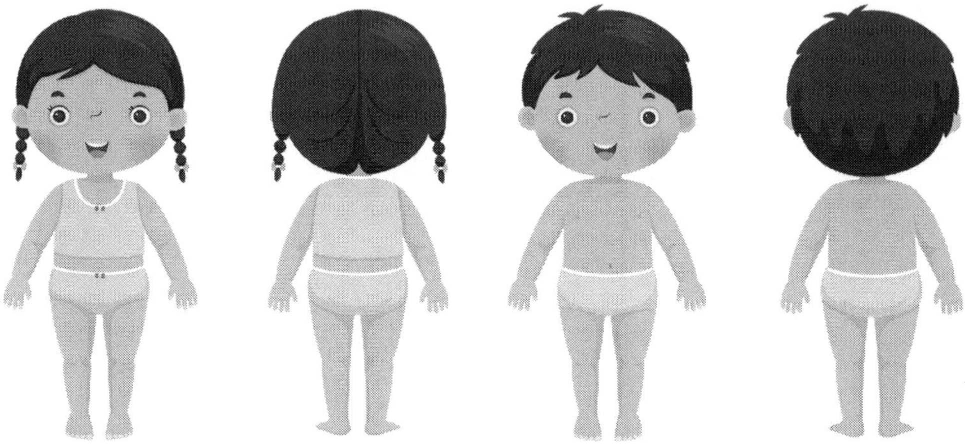

Notes

M T W TH F S SU

Date: / /

	Time	Blood Sugar	Carbs	Insulin	Notes
Breakfast					
Snack					
Lunch					
Snack					
Dinner					
Bedtime					
Night					

M T W TH F S SU Date: / /

Shot Location

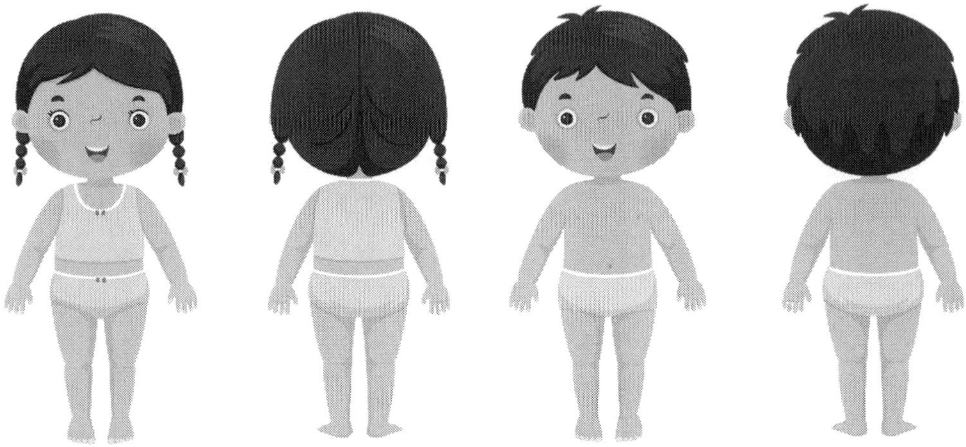

Notes

M T W TH F S SU

Date: / /

	Time	Blood Sugar	Carbs	Insulin	Notes
Breakfast					
Snack					
Lunch					
Snack					
Dinner					
Bedtime					
Night					

M T W TH F S SU Date: / /

Shot Location

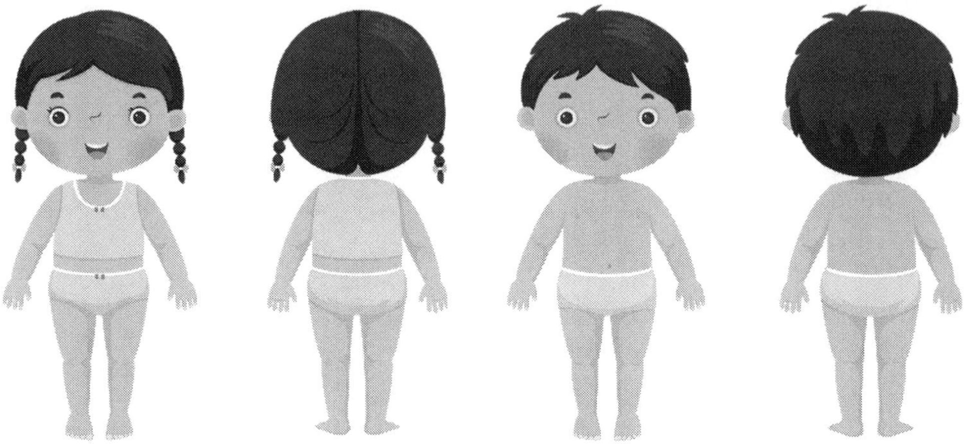

Notes

M T W TH F S SU Date: / /

	Time	Blood Sugar	Carbs	Insulin	Notes
Breakfast					
Snack					
Lunch					
Snack					
Dinner					
Bedtime					
Night					

M T W TH F S SU

Date: / /

Shot Location

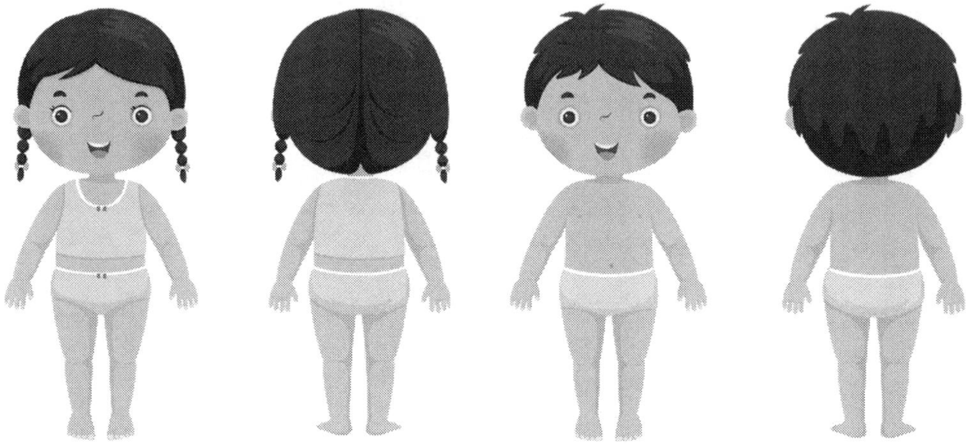

Notes

M T W TH F S SU

Date: / /

	Time	Blood Sugar	Carbs	Insulin	Notes
Breakfast					
Snack					
Lunch					
Snack					
Dinner					
Bedtime					
Night					

M T W TH F S SU Date: / /

Shot Location

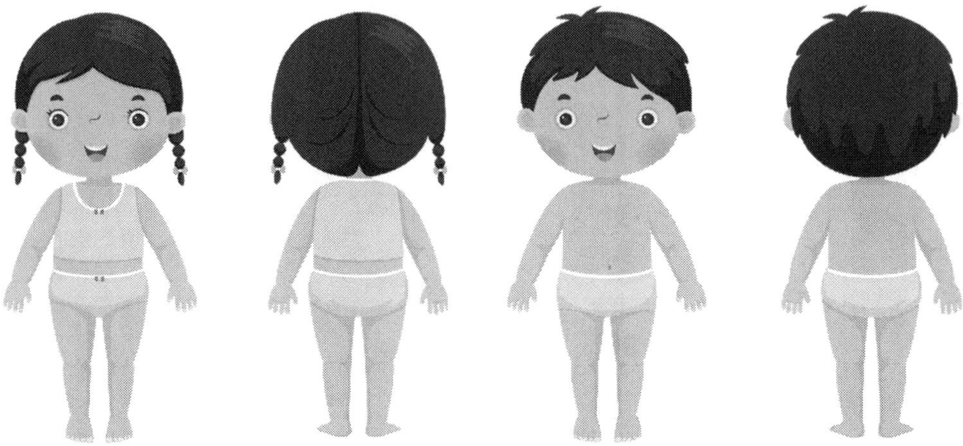

Notes

M T W TH F S SU

Date: / /

	Time	Blood Sugar	Carbs	Insulin	Notes
Breakfast					
Snack					
Lunch					
Snack					
Dinner					
Bedtime					
Night					

M T W TH F S SU Date: / /

Shot Location

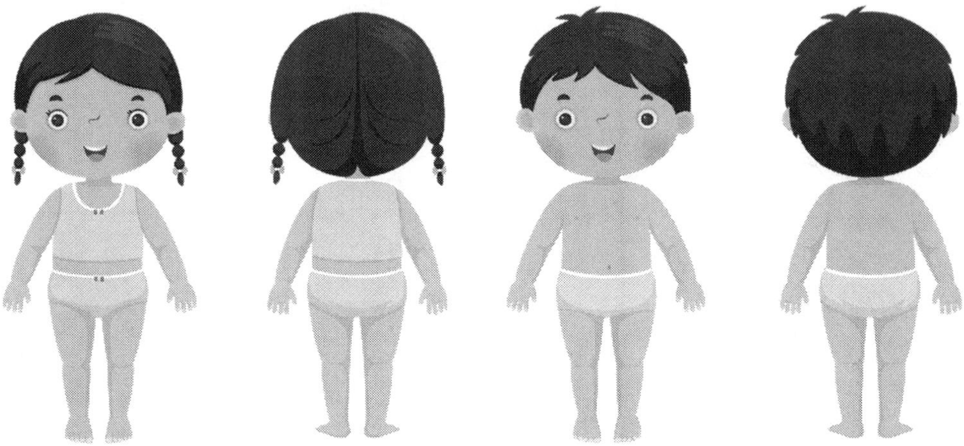

Notes

M T W TH F S SU

Date: / /

	Time	Blood Sugar	Carbs	Insulin	Notes
Breakfast					
Snack					
Lunch					
Snack					
Dinner					
Bedtime					
Night					

M T W TH F S SU Date: / /

Shot Location

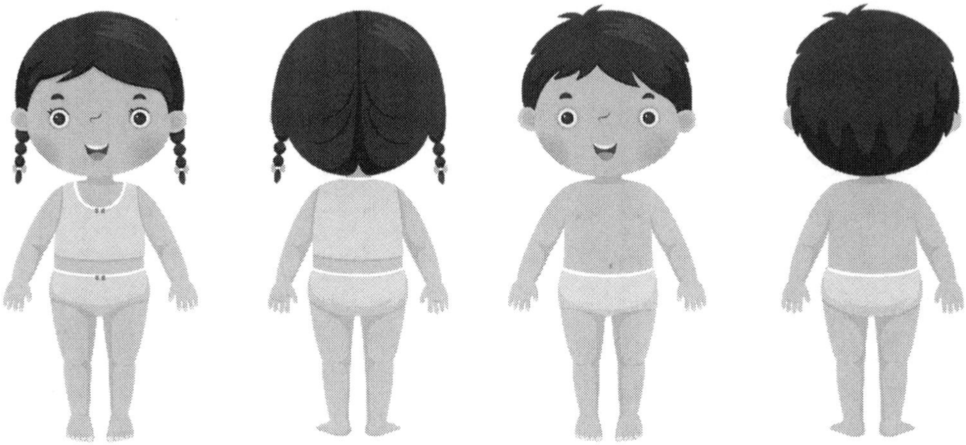

Notes

M T W TH F S SU

Date: / /

	Time	Blood Sugar	Carbs	Insulin	Notes
Breakfast					
Snack					
Lunch					
Snack					
Dinner					
Bedtime					
Night					

M T W TH F S SU Date: / /

Shot Location

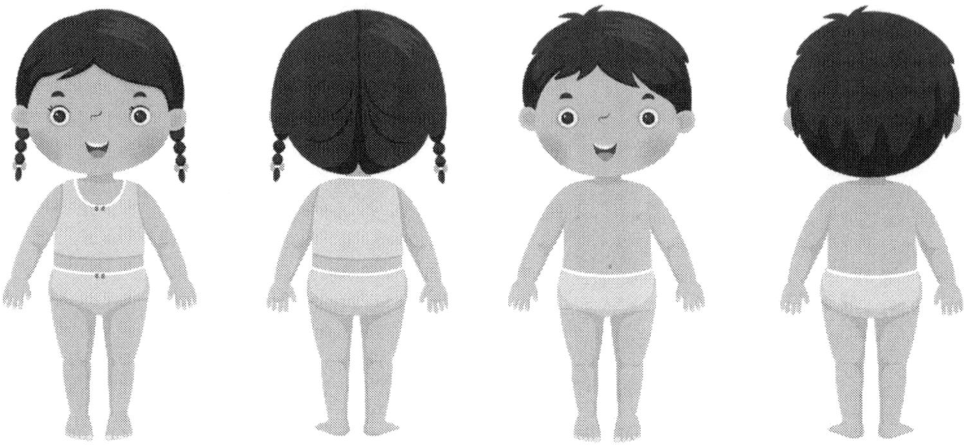

Notes

M T W TH F S SU

Date: / /

	Time	Blood Sugar	Carbs	Insulin	Notes
Breakfast					
Snack					
Lunch					
Snack					
Dinner					
Bedtime					
Night					

M T W TH F S SU Date: / /

Shot Location

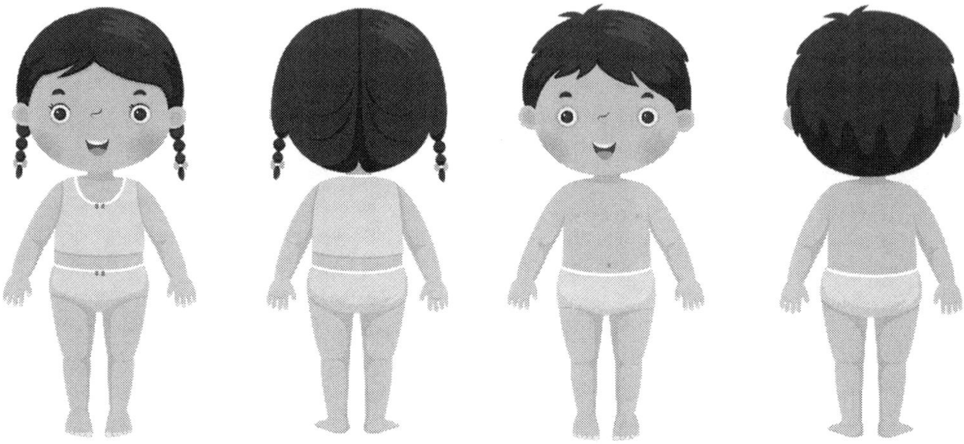

Notes

M T W TH F S SU

Date: / /

	Time	Blood Sugar	Carbs	Insulin	Notes
Breakfast					
Snack					
Lunch					
Snack					
Dinner					
Bedtime					
Night					

M T W TH F S SU Date: / /

Shot Location

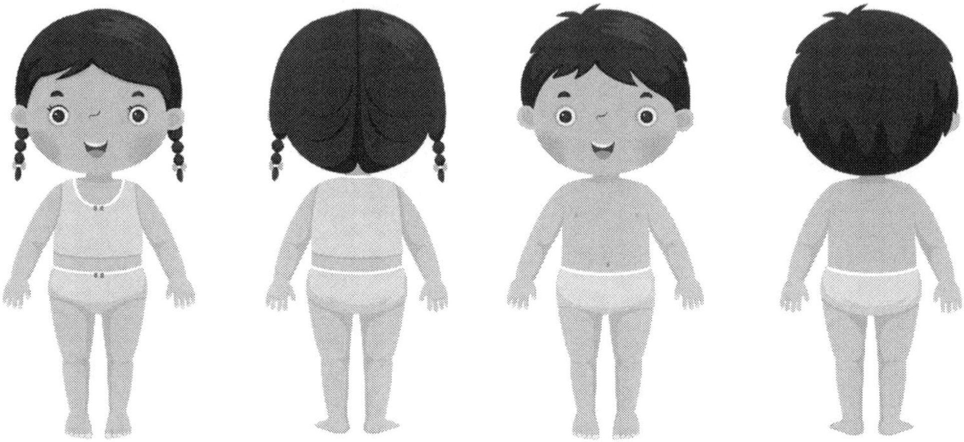

Notes

M T W TH F S SU

Date: / /

	Time	Blood Sugar	Carbs	Insulin	Notes
Breakfast					
Snack					
Lunch					
Snack					
Dinner					
Bedtime					
Night					

M T W TH F S SU Date: / /

Shot Location

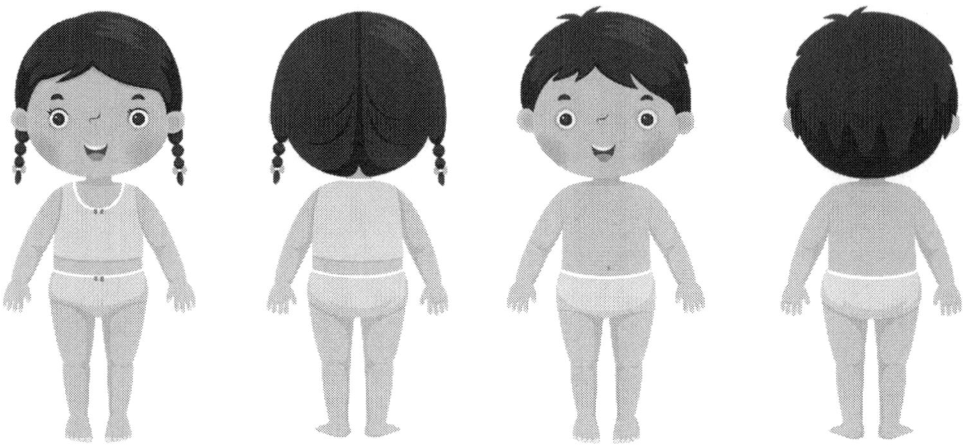

Notes

M T W TH F S SU

Date: / /

	Time	Blood Sugar	Carbs	Insulin	Notes
Breakfast					
Snack					
Lunch					
Snack					
Dinner					
Bedtime					
Night					

M T W TH F S SU Date: / /

Shot Location

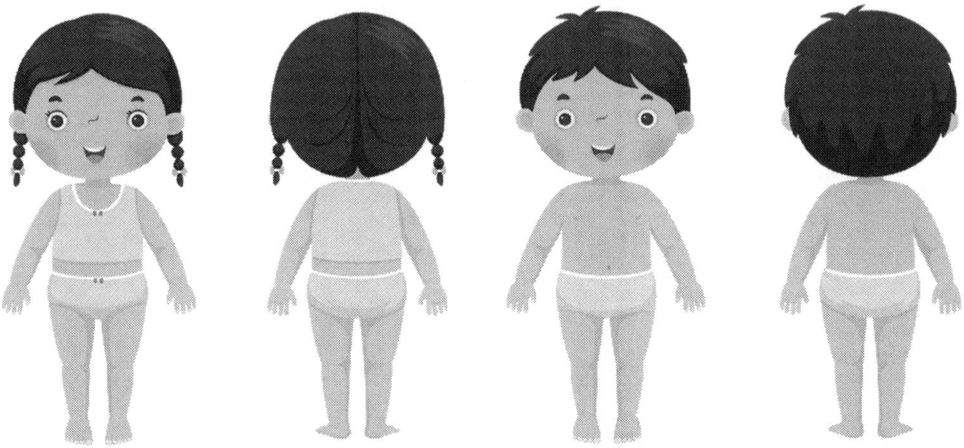

Notes

M T W TH F S SU

Date: / /

	Time	Blood Sugar	Carbs	Insulin	Notes
Breakfast					
Snack					
Lunch					
Snack					
Dinner					
Bedtime					
Night					

M T W TH F S SU Date: / /

Shot Location

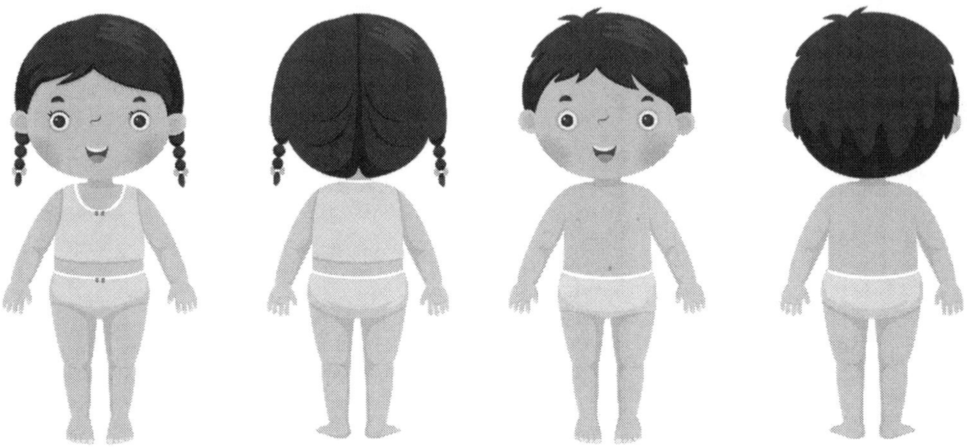

Notes

M T W TH F S SU

Date: / /

	Time	Blood Sugar	Carbs	Insulin	Notes
Breakfast					
Snack					
Lunch					
Snack					
Dinner					
Bedtime					
Night					

M T W TH F S SU Date: / /

Shot Location

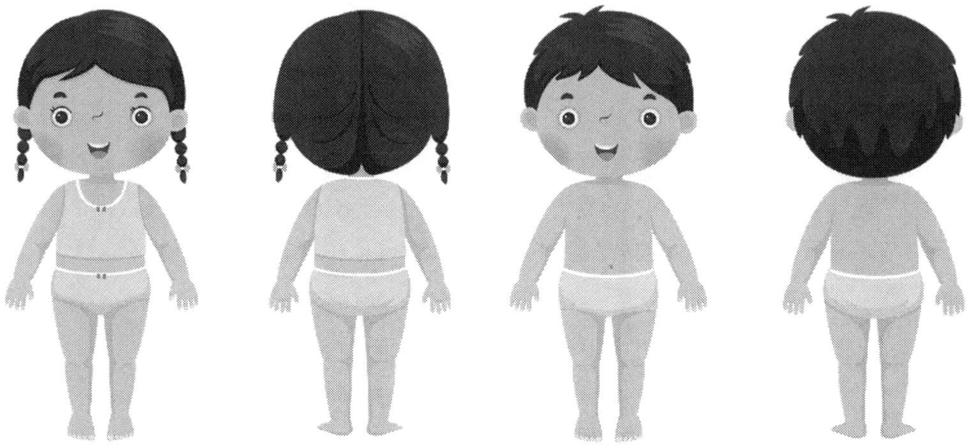

Notes

M T W TH F S SU   Date: / /

	Time	Blood Sugar	Carbs	Insulin	Notes
Breakfast					
Snack					
Lunch					
Snack					
Dinner					
Bedtime					
Night					

M T W TH F S SU

Date: / /

Shot Location

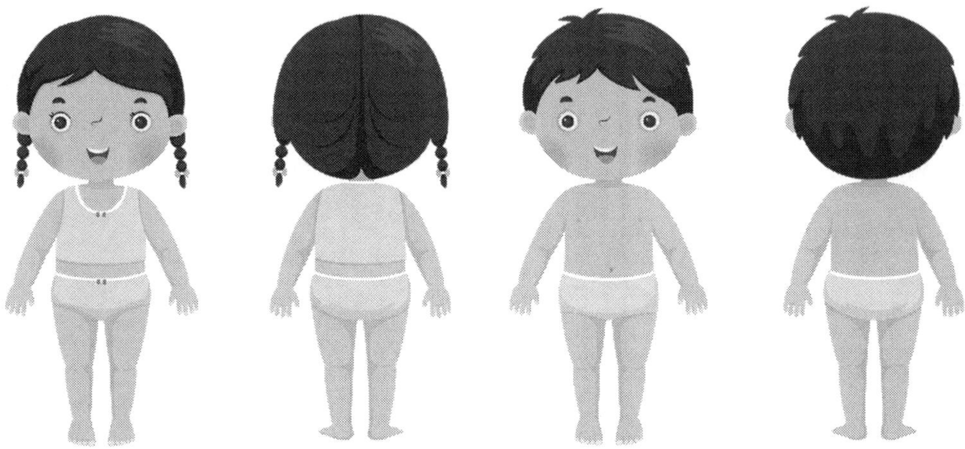

Notes

M T W TH F S SU Date: / /

	Time	Blood Sugar	Carbs	Insulin	Notes
Breakfast					
Snack					
Lunch					
Snack					
Dinner					
Bedtime					
Night					

M T W TH F S SU

Date: / /

Shot Location

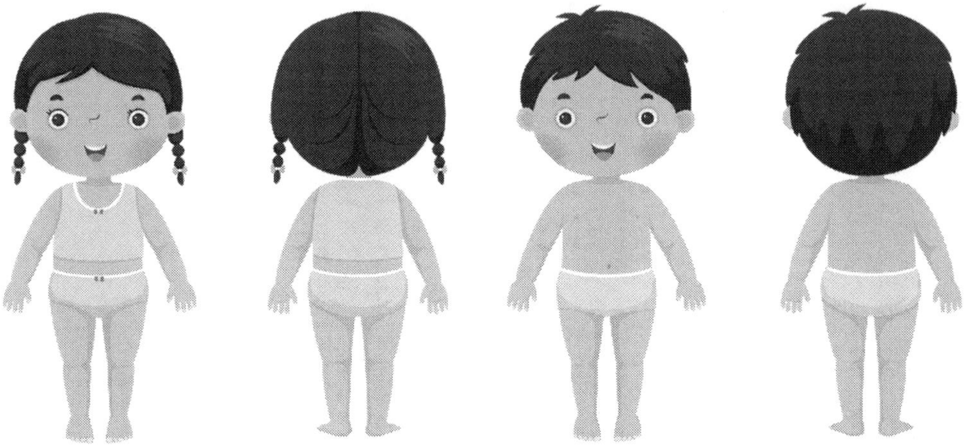

Notes

M T W TH F S SU Date: / /

	Time	Blood Sugar	Carbs	Insulin	Notes
Breakfast					
Snack					
Lunch					
Snack					
Dinner					
Bedtime					
Night					

M T W TH F S SU Date: / /

Shot Location

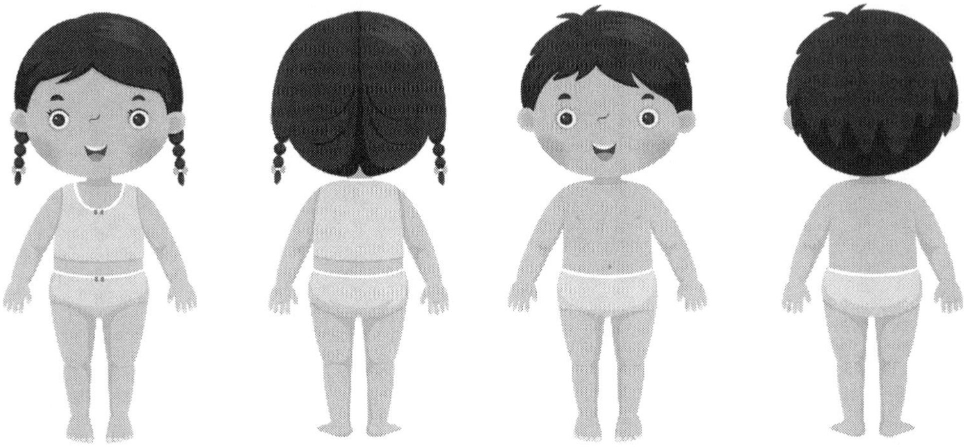

Notes

M T W TH F S SU

Date: / /

	Time	Blood Sugar	Carbs	Insulin	Notes
Breakfast					
Snack					
Lunch					
Snack					
Dinner					
Bedtime					
Night					

M T W TH F S SU Date: / /

Shot Location

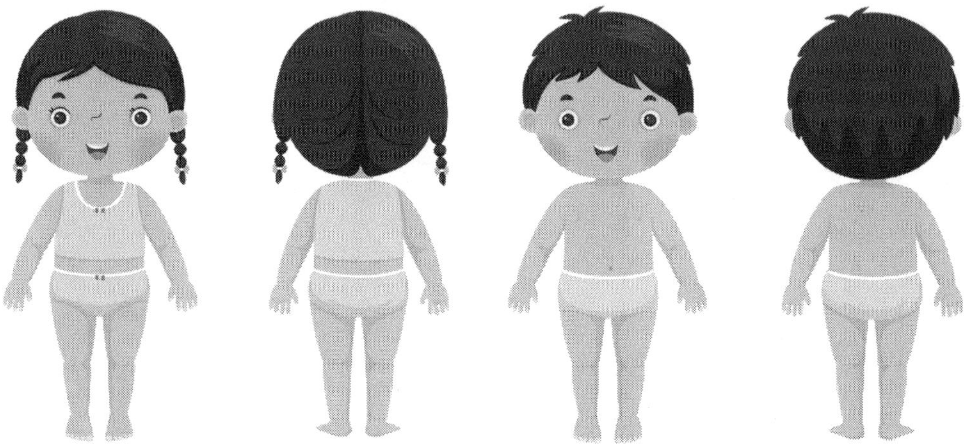

Notes

M T W TH F S SU

Date: / /

	Time	Blood Sugar	Carbs	Insulin	Notes
Breakfast					
Snack					
Lunch					
Snack					
Dinner					
Bedtime					
Night					

M T W TH F S SU Date: / /

Shot Location

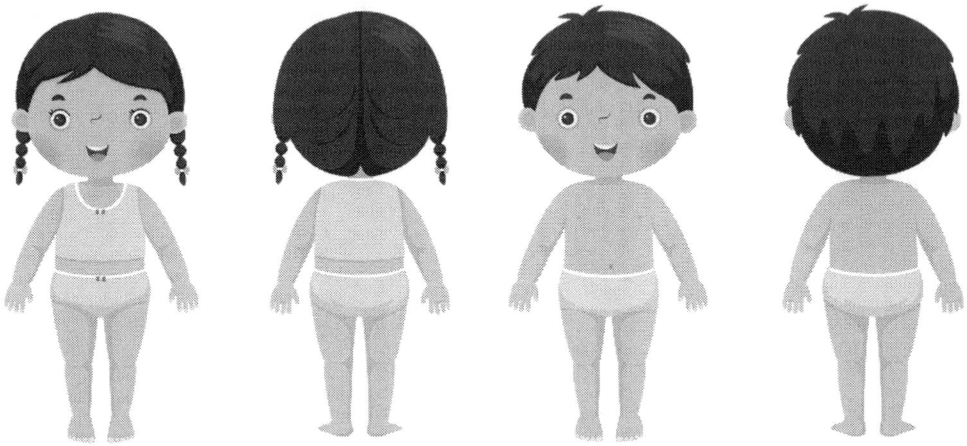

Notes

M T W TH F S SU

Date: / /

	Time	Blood Sugar	Carbs	Insulin	Notes
Breakfast					
Snack					
Lunch					
Snack					
Dinner					
Bedtime					
Night					

M T W TH F S SU Date: / /

Shot Location

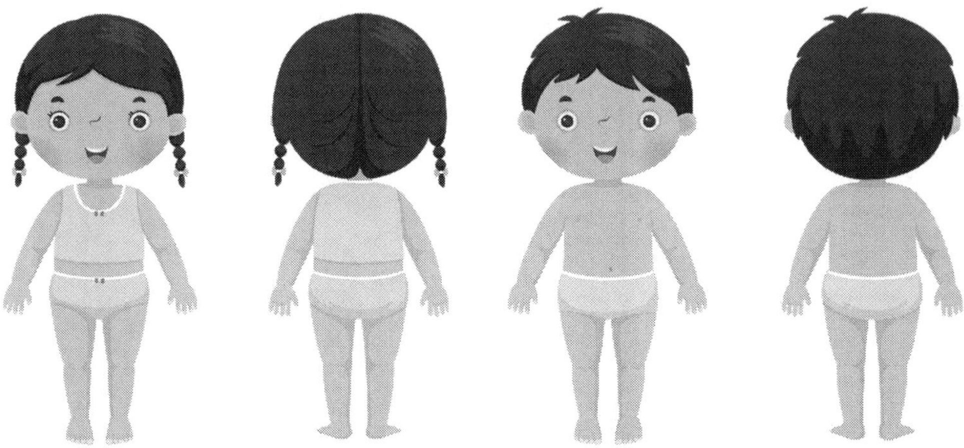

Notes

M T W TH F S SU

Date: / /

	Time	Blood Sugar	Carbs	Insulin	Notes
Breakfast					
Snack					
Lunch					
Snack					
Dinner					
Bedtime					
Night					

M T W TH F S SU Date: / /

Shot Location

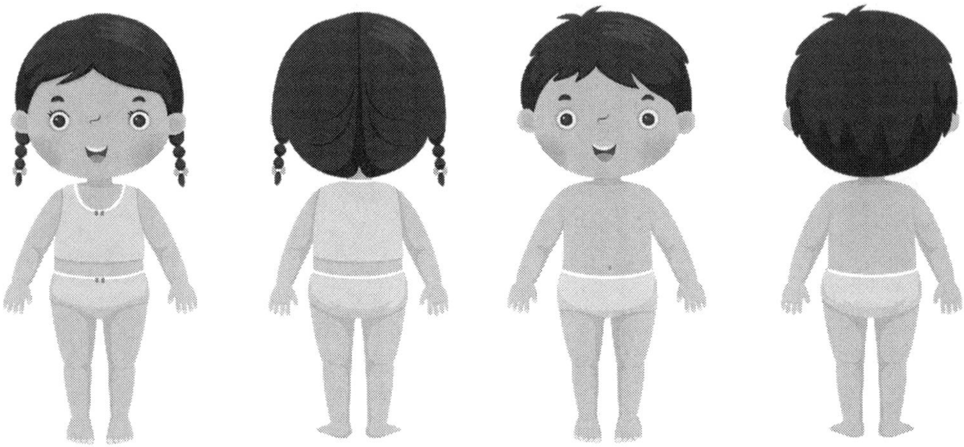

Notes

M T W TH F S SU

Date: / /

	Time	Blood Sugar	Carbs	Insulin	Notes
Breakfast					
Snack					
Lunch					
Snack					
Dinner					
Bedtime					
Night					

M T W TH F S SU Date: / /

Shot Location

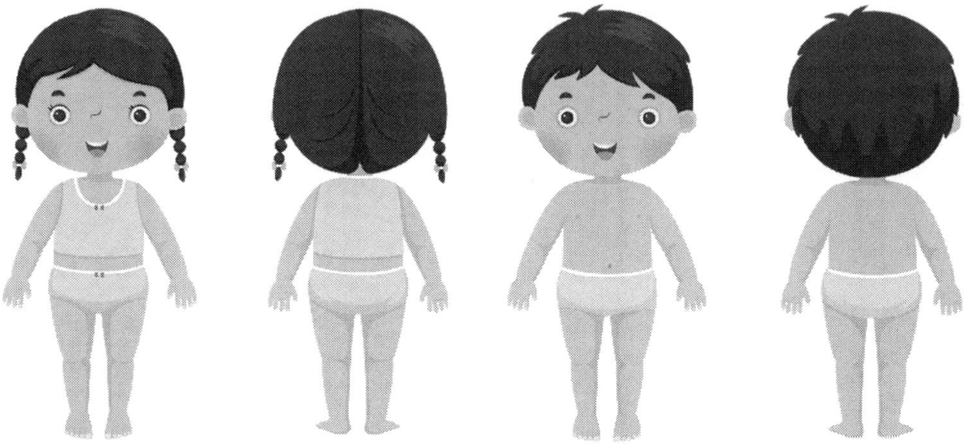

Notes

M T W TH F S SU

Date: / /

	Time	Blood Sugar	Carbs	Insulin	Notes
Breakfast					
Snack					
Lunch					
Snack					
Dinner					
Bedtime					
Night					

M T W TH F S SU

Date: / /

Shot Location

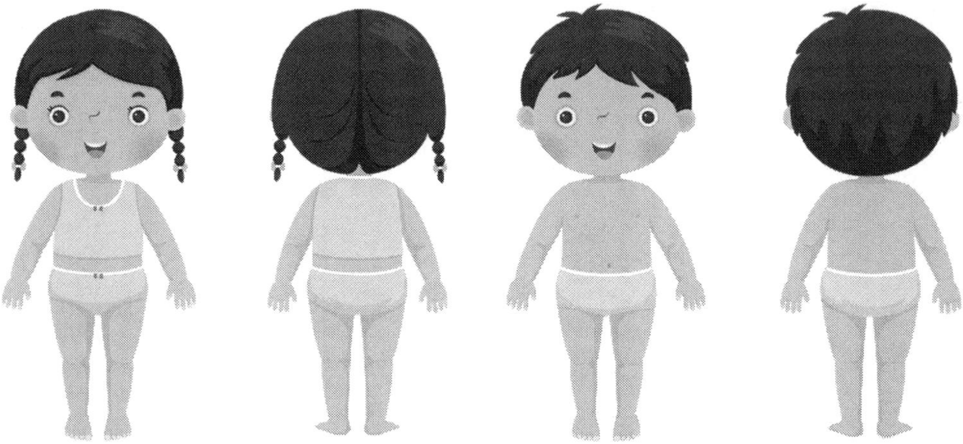

Notes

M T W TH F S SU

Date: / /

	Time	Blood Sugar	Carbs	Insulin	Notes
Breakfast					
Snack					
Lunch					
Snack					
Dinner					
Bedtime					
Night					

M T W TH F S SU

Date: / /

Shot Location

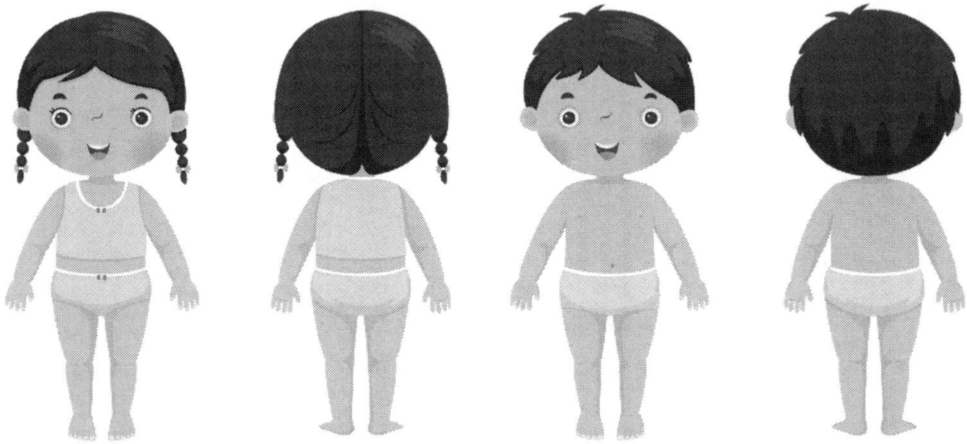

Notes

M T W TH F S SU Date: / /

	Time	Blood Sugar	Carbs	Insulin	Notes
Breakfast					
Snack					
Lunch					
Snack					
Dinner					
Bedtime					
Night					

M T W TH F S SU Date: / /

Shot Location

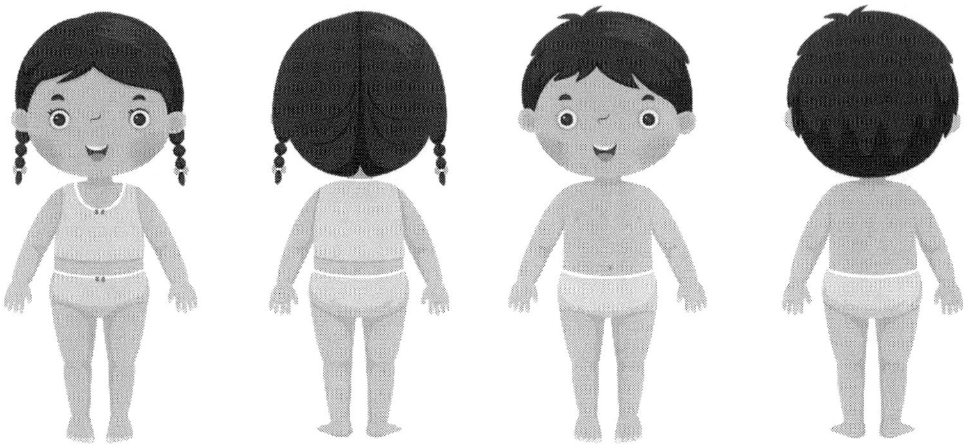

Notes

M T W TH F S SU

Date: / /

	Time	Blood Sugar	Carbs	Insulin	Notes
Breakfast					
Snack					
Lunch					
Snack					
Dinner					
Bedtime					
Night					

M T W TH F S SU Date: / /

Shot Location

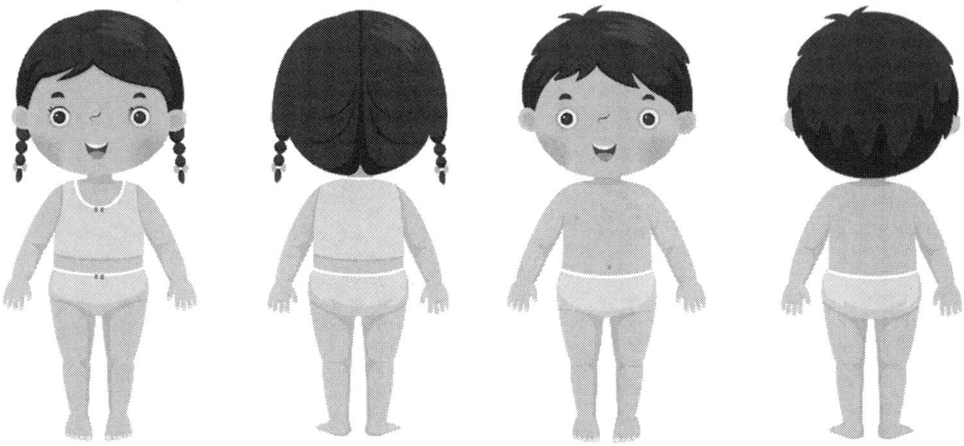

Notes

M T W TH F S SU

Date: / /

	Time	Blood Sugar	Carbs	Insulin	Notes
Breakfast					
Snack					
Lunch					
Snack					
Dinner					
Bedtime					
Night					

M T W TH F S SU Date: / /

Shot Location

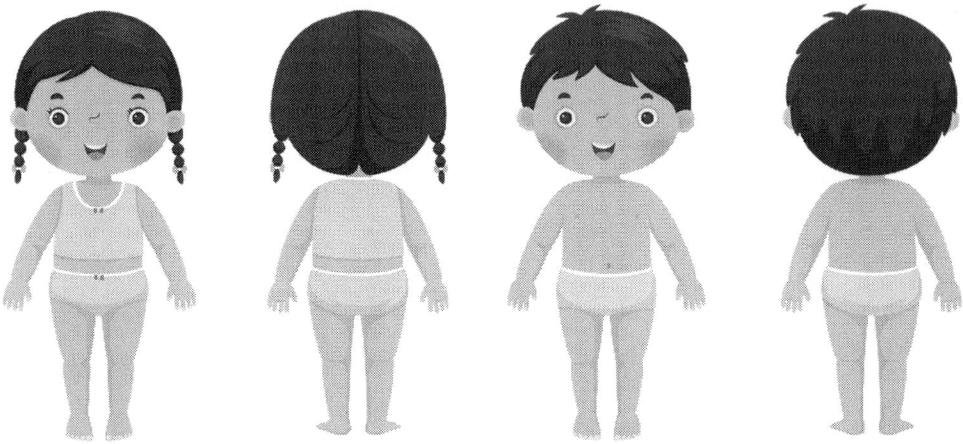

Notes

M T W TH F S SU

Date: / /

	Time	Blood Sugar	Carbs	Insulin	Notes
Breakfast					
Snack					
Lunch					
Snack					
Dinner					
Bedtime					
Night					

M T W TH F S SU

Date: / /

Shot Location

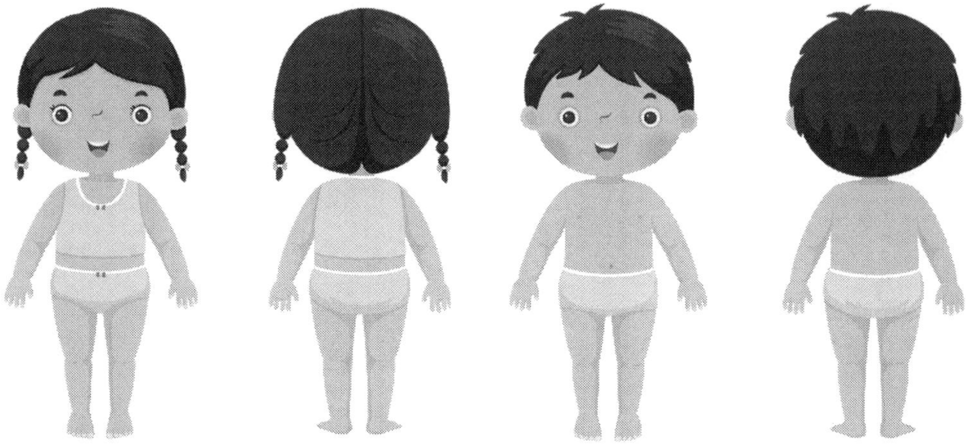

Notes

M T W TH F S SU

Date: / /

	Time	Blood Sugar	Carbs	Insulin	Notes
Breakfast					
Snack					
Lunch					
Snack					
Dinner					
Bedtime					
Night					

M T W TH F S SU Date: / /

Shot Location

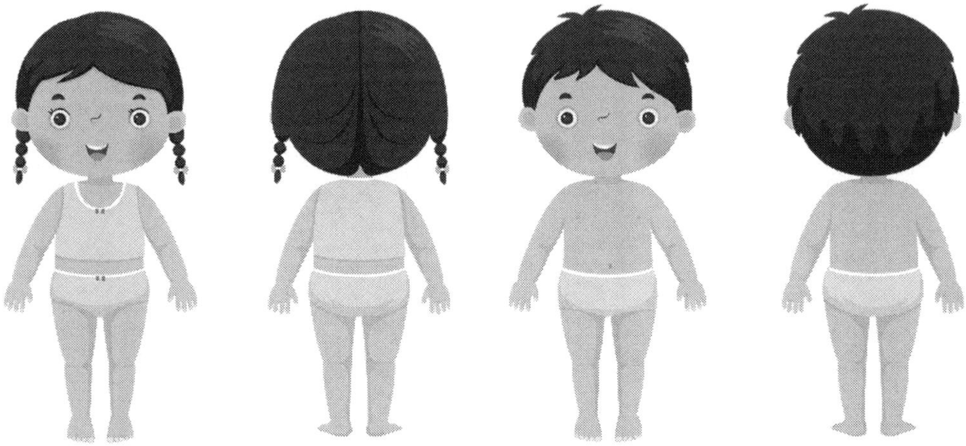

Notes

M T W TH F S SU

Date: / /

	Time	Blood Sugar	Carbs	Insulin	Notes
Breakfast					
Snack					
Lunch					
Snack					
Dinner					
Bedtime					
Night					

Type One Toddler

Made in the USA
Columbia, SC
23 January 2025

52263961R00096